EMERGENCY TOXICOLOGY
Management of Common Poisons

Editor
S.K. Gupta

Associate Editors
S.S. Peshin □ T. Kaleekal □ A. Srivastava □ J. Prakash

Narosa Publishing House
New Delhi   Chennai   Mumbai   Kolkata

EDITOR
S K Gupta
Professor and Head
Department of Pharmacology, and
Chief, National Poisons Information Centre
All India Institute of Medical Sciences
New Delhi-110029, India

ASSOCIATE EDITORS
S.S. Peshin, T. Kaleekal, A. Srivastava and J. Prakash
National Poisons Information Centre
All India Institute of Medical Sciences
New Delhi-110029, India

N A R O S A P U B L I S H I N G H O U S E

22 Daryaganj, Delhi Medical Association Road, New Delhi 110 002
35–36 Greams Road, Thousand Lights, Chennai 600 006
306 Shiv Centre, D.B.C. Sector 17, K.U. Bazar P.O., Navi Mumbai 400 705
2F–2G Shivam Chambers, 53 Syed Amir Ali Avenue, Kolkata 700 019

ISBN 81-7319-474-2

Published by N.K. Mehra for Narosa Publishing House, 22 Daryaganj,
Delhi Medical Association Road, New Delhi 110 002 and printed at
Chaman Enterprises, New Delhi 110 002, India.

Preface

Poisoning is recognized as an important health problem in many developed countries but it is ill defined in developing countries including India. In our country, one of the largest industrialized nations, assessment of the problem is of paramount importance as there is no epidemiological data on actual incidence of poisoning due to lack of systematic reporting to a central agency. In developed countries, the problem of poisoning has been tackled to a certain extent by executing Poisons Control Programmes which provide the framework for prevention and management of poisoning. The Poisons Information Centre is an essential component of such a programme which among its multiple roles, includes the provision of clinical and toxicological information and its dissemination to treating physicians, paramedical personnel, government agencies, industries and community at large. In India, the need for such a programme was recognized and as a part of the activity the National Poisons Information Centre (NPIC) was set up in the Department of Pharmacology at the All India Institute of Medical Sciences, New Delhi in 1995. The Centre which is first of its kind in the country provides tailor made information and advice on the management of various poisonings round-the-clock, 7 days a week on telephone, fax and e-mail.

The efficient management of poisoning patients depends on provision of good supportive care, knowledge of symptomatology of various chemical agents, diagnosis and antidotal therapy to be employed. From our experience at NPIC, it has been found that inadequate knowledge about trade names especially of pesticides, exact management guidelines, antidotes, their dosages and availability are responsible for poor prognosis of these patients. With this idea, we have designed this manual which is a brief set of guidelines for medical professionals and paramedical personnels to aid them in managing cases of poisoning. Though poisoning can be caused by a wide variety of chemical agents, an effort has been made to include only those agents which are commonly consumed, on the basis of our experience at NPIC. The manual provides updated toxicological information derived from published medical and toxicological texts on commonly encountered drugs, pesticides, household products, industrial chemicals, environmental toxins, heavy metals and an array of miscellaneous agents. Various uses, mechanism of toxicity, toxic dose, diagnosis, clinical features, monitoring and both the prehospital and hospital management have been dealt with in a lucid manner. The trade names especially of pesticides have been included which may provide a ready reference for knowing the composition of a product. Toxic doses wherever available have been incorporated. A chapter on common therapeutic drugs and antidotes, their indications and doses has been compiled at the back to avoid repetition in the text.

I deeply acknowledge the dedicated and sincere efforts put in by the staff of the National Poisons Information Centre in compiling information on management of various poisonings. On behalf of all authors, I record thanks to Mrs. Rita Sharma, Computer Operator for excellent presentation of the book.

I hope this book will serve as a ready reference to any hospital or health care facility managing poisoning cases.

S.K. GUPTA
Editor

Contents

General Principles in the Management of Poisoning

Poisoning is an emergency situation requiring immediate medical attention. The poisoned patient needs to be evaluated thoroughly and general principles of management are to be followed. The goals to be achieved include recognition of poisoning, identification and prediction of toxicity of the poison and assessment of severity of poisoning. The initial steps include clinical assessment of the condition of the patient and maintenance of basic vital functions (BP, ECG, pupillary size, body temperature and neurological functions). Efforts should be directed at obtaining an accurate history of the poisoning case. All baseline laboratory investigations need to be carried out. Quantitative analysis of toxin in blood, urine, aspirate may help in the diagnosis and prognosis. Good supportive care superceeds all other measures and includes the care of the airway, breathing and circulation.

Decontamination procedures include removal of contaminated clothes, shoes, washing of patient's skin etc., taking due precautions by wearing aprons, gloves and face masks. Dilution with water or demulcents like milk may help in reducing gastrointestinal irritation, however excessive amounts should be avoided. Prevention of further absorption of the toxin in the body is achieved by active removal of toxic substance from the body by inducing emesis. Emesis can be induced either by mechanical (tickling the back of the throat by fingers) or chemical means (using syrup of ipecac). One of the important requirements of this procedure is that the patient must be conscious. Emesis is contraindicated in ingestion of corrosives, low viscosity and high volatility petroleum distillates, patients showing altered sensorium and those at risk of developing convulsions. Emesis is also contraindicated in third trimester of pregnancy. Activated charcoal may be administered following emesis.

Gastric lavage with water, normal saline, sodium bicarbonate, potassium permanganate, calcium salts etc., after taking appropriate precautions like endotracheal intubation in unconscious patients and controlling seizures is helpful in removing toxins. Gastric lavage is reported to be most effective within an hour of ingestion. The contraindications of gastric lavage include ingestion of hydrocarbons, acids/alkalies etc. It should not be used on a routine basis.

The adsorption of the ingested poison is reduced by using adsorbents like activated charcoal, cholestyramine, Fuller's earth, bentonite etc. Sorbitol or a saline cathartic should accompany charcoal administration in order to enhance gut motility and to possibly increase toxin elimination. Administration of multiple doses of a cathartic may impair fluid and electrolyte balance and is therefore not recommended in infants and children. Cathartic administration is also contraindicated in case of absent bowel sounds, abdominal trauma or surgery, intestinal perforation or obstruction, volume depletion, hypotension, electrolyte imbalance, corrosive ingestion etc.

Seizures may be managed by benzodiazepines or phenytoin and phenobarbital. Efforts should always be directed towards increasing elimination of toxins from body which can be done by using both invasive and non invasive procedures. Non invasive procedures include multiple dose charcoal therapy and forced diuresis. The invasive elimination methods include peritoneal and hemodialysis, hemoperfusion and plasma exchange etc. The prompt administration of antidotes to a poisoned patient is of vital importance in life saving. The purpose is to reduce toxicity and improve prognosis.

1. Drugs

Nonsteroidal anti-inflammatory drugs

Nonsteroidal anti-inflammatory drugs (NSAIDs) are the frequently sold over-the-counter drugs. Their popularity is widespread all over the world on account of their excellent anti-inflammatory, analgesic and antipyretic properties. Despite their varied chemical nature, they are very similar in their clinical efficacy and are available as tablets and capsules, sustained release tablets and capsules, suspensions and ophthalmic solutions. They are also available in combination usually with paracetamol. NSAIDs are indicated for the treatment of ankylosing spondylitis, fever, corneal ulcers, seasonal allergic conjunctivitis, headache, prophylaxis of myocardial infarction, degenerative joint diseases (osteoarthritis, rheumatoid arthritis etc.), acute musculoskeletal disorders, tendonitis and unstable angina etc.

Mechanism of toxicity

All NSAIDs cause local gastric irritation and inhibit the synthesis of cytoprotective prostaglandins in the gastric mucosa (as a result weakening of GI mucosal barrier) leading partly to GI symptoms. NSAIDs induced GI bleeding occurs because of inhibition of TXA_2 production in platelets resulting in prolongation of bleeding time. Inhibition of PGE_2 and PGI_2 in the renal arteries causes salt and water retention.

Toxic dose

Significant toxicity occurs after acute ingestion of 5–10 times the usual therapeutic dose of NSAIDs. Ibuprofen is relatively safe compared with other members of its group. Symptoms usually do not occur at the dose of 100 mg/kg body weight. Life threatening symptoms occur at the dose of 400 mg/kg. The mild toxic dose in children is 200–400 mg/kg. Severe toxicity occurs in children if the dose exceeds 400 mg/kg. The adult toxic dose of piroxicam is 300–600 mg. Severe multisystem organ toxicity has been observed with 100 mg of piroxicam in a 2 year old child. Severe toxicity occurs with the ingestion of 300–500 mg/kg of sodium salicylate. Death has been reported with the ingestion of 10–30 g. Ingestion of 1.5 g of diclofenac produces toxic symptoms. Death is reported within 2 days after acute ingestion of 5 g of diclofenac in a young male. The toxicity of indomethacin is less as compared with oxyphenbutazone and phenylbutazone. Renal failure is reported in a preterm infant with symptomatic patent ductus arteriosus who received 100 fold overdose of indomethacin. The toxic doses of naproxen and sulindac are 10 g and 12 g, respectively, in adults. Mefenamic acid and meclofenamate are relatively more toxic than other NSAIDs. Severe symptoms have been observed in an adult female with acute ingestion of 22.5 g of mefenamic acid. Oxyphenbutazone and phenylbutazone are more toxic in overdose. More than 4 g of phenylbutazone is associated with severe toxicity. Acute toxic dose of oxaprozin, nimesulide, meloxicam, celecoxib, rofecoxib and tolmetin is not known as yet.

Clinical features

- Acute overdose mostly causes lethargy, GI upset (nausea, vomiting, abdominal pain, diarrhea), metabolic acidosis, respiratory alkalosis, electrolyte disturbance, hematuria, sodium and water retention, pulmonary edema etc.
- Severe overdose may cause hypotension, coma, respiratory depression, GI bleeding or acute renal insufficiency rarely.
- Risk of kidney damage is similar with both selective (COX-2) and non-selective cyclooxygenase (COX-1 and COX-2) inhibitors.
- Hepatic necrosis is also reported.
- Seizures are reported most commonly after mefenamic acid overdose but may rarely occur after severe overdose of other NSAIDs also.
- Nimesulide, meloxicam, celecoxib, rofecoxib have lesser potential for upper GI toxicity compared with conventional NSAIDs.
- Severe toxicity of piroxicam overdose produces hyponatremia, hypocalcemia, thrombocytopenia, hematuria, prolongation of prothrombin time and rarely pulmonary edema.
- In addition to general toxic features of NSAIDs, severe toxicity of sodium salicylate overdose also produces, hyperglycemia/hypoglycemia, fever, oliguria, dehydration, renal failure, irritability, disorientation and confusion progressing to coma and death. Death occurs due to respiratory insufficiency and cardiovascular collapse.
- Life threatening symptoms of diclofenac overdose are loss of consciousness, increased intracranial pressure and aspiration pneumonitis.
- Unsteadiness, blurred vision, diarrhea, GI upset and bleeding, headache, agitation, incoherence, confusion, drowsiness and coma are reported in flurbiprofen overdose.
- Tinnitus, confusion, disorientation, restlessness and agitation are also reported with indomethacin.
- Hepatitis has been reported with sulindac in children.

Diagnosis
Diagnosis is based on history of exposure. NSAIDs usually produce mild and nonspecific symptoms.

Laboratory/Monitoring
- Monitor complete blood count (CBC), electrolytes, calcium, magnesium, glucose, BUN, creatinine, liver transaminases and prothrombin time (PT).
- Carry out urinalysis.

Management

Pre-hospital

- Induce emesis with syrup of ipecac as early as possible (preferably within few minutes of ingestion). Do not induce emesis in mefenamic acid intoxication or ibuprofen ingestion of more than 400 mg/kg.
- Administer activated charcoal within 1 hr. of ingestion.

Hospital

- Treatment is supportive and symptomatic.
- Maintain the airway and assist ventilation if necessary. Administer supplemental oxygen.
- Treat seizures with anticonvulsants. Control recurrent seizures with phenobarbital.
- Perform gastric lavage within one hour after massive overdose. Gastric lavage is not necessary if charcoal can be given immediately. Multiple dose activated charcoal is useful in enhancing elimination.
- Treat coma and hypotension.
- Give antacids or sucralfate for GI irritation. Replace fluid losses with IV fluids.
- Vitamin K1 for elevated prothrombin time (due to hypoprothrombinemia).
- Hemodialysis is unlikely to enhance elimination, however, it may be useful if oliguric renal failure occurs.
- Peritoneal dialysis and forced diuresis are not effective. However, forced diuresis has been found effective in diclofenac overdose.
- There is no specific antidote for NSAIDs poisoning.

Paracetamol

Paracetamol (PCM) is a nonsteroidal anti-inflammatory drug (p-amino phenol derivative). It is available alone as tablets, syrups, suspensions, injectable drops and in combination (tablets, capsules, suspensions) usually with one or more of the drugs like ibuprofen, diclofenac, phenylbutazone, chlormezanone, oxyphenbutazone, dextropropoxyphene, pentazocine, metoclopramide, dicyclomine etc. It is mainly used as an analgesic and antipyretic agent. It has weak anti-inflammatory property at therapeutic doses which makes it unsuitable for use in inflammatory conditions.

Mechanism of toxicity
Neither the parent compound nor its metabolites are toxic, however, a small fraction of it undergoes cytochrome P-450 mediated N-hydroxylation to form N-acetylbenzoquinoneimine. In overdose, increased formation of this reactive intermediate depletes the hepatic stores of glutathione leading to hepatic necrosis. Intracellular accumulation of Ca^{2+}, activation of Ca^{2+} dependent endonuclease and resultant DNA fragmentation, at least in part, play a role in paracetamol mediated hepatotoxicity.

Toxic dose
Liver toxicity is likely to occur with the oral ingestion of 140 mg/kg of PCM in adults. A single acute overdose of 10–15 g of the drug is potentially fatal. The risk of toxicity increases in chronic alcoholics and in patients chronically taking INH, rifampicin or both presumably because of induction of liver microsomal enzymes and impairment of glutathione synthesis and consequently increased formation of toxic metabolites of PCM. Children are less susceptible to acute overdose effects as compared with adults. Gilbert's disease is also one of the risk factors for paracetamol poisoning.

Clinical features
Clinical manifestations occur in the following stages:

- Stage I (0.5–24 hrs.) is an early stage characterized by GI symptoms (nausea, vomiting, anorexia, diarrhea), pallor, diaphoresis and malaise.
- Stage II (24–48 hrs.) is characterized by right upper quadrant abdominal pain, pain in flanks, hematuria and metabolic acidosis. Sometimes acute renal failure occurs with or without liver damage. Acute pancreatitis is also seen. Prolongation of prothrombin time, bilirubin and elevation in transaminase levels indicate hepatic necrosis.
- Stage III (48–96 hrs.) shows massive liver damage leading to hepatic failure, encephalopathy, renal insufficiency and myocardial damage.
- Stage IV is the recovery stage occurring one week post ingestion.
- Death occurs due to hepatic and renal failure.

Diagnosis
It is based on history of exposure and quantitative estimation of plasma paracetamol levels.

Laboratory/Monitoring

- Monitor 4 hrs. post ingestion plasma paracetamol levels and predict the severity of toxicity with the help of paracetamol nomogram [time in hrs. after paracetamol ingestion vs. plasma/serum paracetamol concentration (μg/ml)].
- Perform liver function tests (SGOT, SGPT, total bilirubin and INR or

PT) in patients suspected to have toxic paracetamol levels immediately on admission in the hospital and daily for 3 days or until levels begin to return to normal. If significant abnormality in LFT is seen, then monitor creatinine, BUN, electrolytes, glucose, hemoglobin, hematocrit, amylase and ECG.

Management

Pre-hospital

- Induce emesis with syrup of ipecac within 30 min. of exposure.
- Lay patient on left side to prevent aspiration.
- Administer activated charcoal.

Hospital

- Provide oxygenation and ventilatory support if required.
- Control spontaneous vomiting by metoclopramide.
- Perform gastric lavage preferably within 4 hrs. post ingestion, however it has been found to be effective upto 6 hrs. post ingestion.
- Administer activated charcoal, IV fluids and manage metabolic acidosis with sodium bicarbonate.
- Hemoperfusion, though effective, is generally not indicated.
- Massive hepatic failure may necessitate liver transplantation.
- N-acetylcysteine (NAC) is the specific antidote.

Carbamazepine

Carbamazepine is an antiepileptic drug belonging to the class of iminostilbene. It is available as tablets, sustained release tablets, retard tablets and controlled release tablets. It is useful in temporal lobe epilepsies and psychomotor epilepsies. It is also used in trigeminal and glossopharyngeal neuralgia, bipolar affective disorders, aggression and diabetes incipidus.

Mechanism of toxicity

Structurally and pharmacologically, carbamazepine resembles tricyclic antidepressants and meprobamate. In overdose, it thus causes anticholinergic and cardiovascular features.

Toxic dose

Acute ingestion of >10 mg/kg of carbamazepine is likely to be associated with toxicity. Serious toxicity occurs with the ingestion of 50 mg/kg. With ingestion upto 20–30 g no deaths have been reported. Offenders have survived after ingestion of 10 g (6 year old child) and 5 g (3 year old child) of carbamazepine. The metabolism of carbamazepine may be inhibited by concomitant administration of propoxyphene, erythromycin, fluovoxamine,

MAO-inhibitors and lithium, putting the patient at risk of developing toxicity with usual therapeutic doses of carbamazepine. Delayed toxicity is observed with carbamazepine due to delayed gastric emptying.

Clinical features

- Mild toxicity is manifested as drowsiness, slurred speech, nystagmus, dystonic reactions, hallucinations, nausea, vomiting, hyponatremia, mydriasis and decreased GI motility.
- Severe toxicity may lead to coma, seizures, respiratory depression, arrhythmias, decreased myocardial contractility, pulmonary edema and hypotension.
- Elevated liver enzymes, oliguria and bullous skin eruption are observed rarely.

Diagnosis

Diagnosis is based on history of exposure. There is no single characteristic feature of overdose. Ataxia, stupor, tachycardia and serum carbamazepine levels are the diagnostic criteria for carbamazepine overdose.

Laboratory/Monitoring

- Monitor carbamazepine levels. The maximum plasma concentration of carbamazepine is reached at 72 hrs. post ingestion.
- There is no perfect correlation between plasma carbamazepine concentration and clinical features.
- Monitor CBC, glucose, electrolytes, arterial blood gases and ECG.

Management

Pre-hospital

- Induce vomiting as early as possible after ingestion, with syrup of ipecac.
- Administer activated charcoal.

Hospital

- Treatment is supportive and symptomatic.
- Perform gastric lavage even when more than 4 hrs. have elapsed.
- Administer repeat dose activated charcoal.
- Monitor cardiac status and correct electrolyte imbalance.
- Treat seizures with anticonvulsants. Control recurrent seizures with phenobarbital. Delayed absorption can cause a relapse on 2nd and 3rd day.
- Charcoal hemoperfusion is highly effective in life-threatening

ventricular arrhythmias refractory to standard therapy or status epilepticus.
- Hemodialysis and peritoneal dialysis are not effective.
- Flumazenil has been found to be effective in a few cases.
- There is no specific antidote.

Benzodiazepines

Benzodiazepines (BDZs) are the frequently prescribed antianxiety drugs. They are available as tablets, capsules, suspension and as injectables and are indicated for the symptomatic relief of anxiety, seizures and sleep disorders, alcohol/hypnotic withdrawal. They are also used as pre-anaesthetic medications and as muscle relaxants. Benzodiazepines have replaced barbiturates in the treatment of anxiety and insomnia as they are more safe, effective and produce less tolerance and physical dependence when used chronically. They have minimal cytochrome P-450 induction ability.

Mechanism of toxicity

Binding of BDZs to its receptors (GABA$_A$ but not GABA$_B$) causes GABA$_A$ receptor mediated increased in Cl$^-$ conductance, generalized depression of spinal reflexes and reticular activating system leading to coma and respiratory arrest in massive overdose. Whether BDZs enhance the inhibitory actions of other neurotransmitters also, remains to be elucidated.

Toxic dose

BDZs have very wide therapeutic window. They are associated with low toxicity unless ingested with other CNS depressants especially ethanol. In high doses CNS and respiratory depression is seen. Elderly are highly susceptible to the CNS and respiratory depressant effects of BDZs. Deaths are rare from BDZ overdose alone. Oral ingestion of alprazolam 20–60mg produces mild lethargy and combativeness. Minor toxicity is observed with 500 mg to 2 g of diazepam. Overdose toxicity of flunitrazepam is similar to or more than other BDZs. Toxic dose in children is 0.26–0.29 mg/kg body weight. Fatal dose of lorazepam in adults and children is approximately 1.85 g and 500–600 mg respectively. However surprisingly, drowsiness and ataxia have been reported in a 6 year old child 2 hrs. after ingestion of 30 mg of lorazepam. Severe toxicity has been reported after ingestion of 900 mg of oxazepam in an adult. Adult lethal dose of triazolam is 12.5 mg. Its toxic dose in children is 0.06–0.07 mg/kg.

Clinical features

- Acute BDZ overdose is manifested by varying degree of CNS depression (drowsiness to coma).
- Mild symptoms are drowsiness, ataxia, lethargy, confusion and slurred speech.

- Drowsiness, agitation and ataxia are more common in children.
- Hypotonia is rare but a severe poisoning symptom in children.
- Most obtunded patients become arousable within 12–36 hrs. following overdose.
- Specific features of diazepam overdose are somnolence, confusion, dysarthria, diplopia, diminished reflexes and coma. Bullous skin eruption is a rare toxicity.
- Grade I coma with absent deep tendon reflexes are reported in oxazepam toxicity.
- Respiratory arrest is more likely with triazolam, alprazolam and midazolam as compared with other BDZs.
- Hostility and hallucinations are reported with IV overdose of midazolam. Emergence of delirium is reported in children.

Diagnosis

Diagnosis is based on history of exposure. Rule out the toxic ingestion of sedative hypnotics, antidepressants, psychopharmacological agents, narcotics etc.

Laboratory/Monitoring

- Plasma/serum levels of BDZs may be available but are not usually clinically useful in emergency management.
- Monitor glucose, arterial blood gases, creatinine, electrolytes and creatinine phosphokinase (CPK), urinalysis, BUN and ECG.
- Perform CT (head), lumber puncture and chest X-ray if necessary.
- Monitor PCM, aspirin and ethanol to detect occult ingestion.
- Immunoassays and HPLC may be useful in detection of certain benzodiazepines.

Management

Pre-hospital

- Induce emesis with syrup of ipecac within few minutes of exposure. Avoid emesis in patients who have ingested ultrashort acting BDZs such as triazolam.
- Administer activated charcoal.

Hospital

- Treatment is supportive and symptomatic.
- Perform gastric lavage in massive overdose preferably within one hour of ingestion.
- Administer activated charcoal.
- Regularly monitor vital signs especially respiration and provide assisted ventilation if required.

- Correct hypotension by infusing IV fluids and vasopressors.
- Role of forced diuresis is not well established, however, it has been found to improve symptoms in diazepam poisoning.
- Hemodialysis is not effective.
- Manage initial withdrawal symptoms with phenobarbital/diazepam, then reduce the dose by about 10% per day of initial dose required to control symptoms.
- Flumazenil is the specific antidote. However, it should be administered only to severely poisoned patients.

Barbiturates

Barbiturates, the derivatives of thiobarbituric acid were widely used sedative-hypnotics till 1960s. However, they have been largely replaced by BDZs now-a-days. The popularity of barbiturates has decreased because of their adverse effects, high incidence of drug dependence, withdrawal symptoms on sudden stoppage and their abuse potential.

The major groups of barbiturates are shown in Table 1.

Table 1. Major groups of barbiturates

Long acting (6–12 hrs.)[1]	Short acting (2–3 hrs.)[2]
Phenobarbital, Mephobarbitone	Secobarbitone, Pentobarbitone
Barbitone, Primidone	Hexobarbitone
Intermediate acting (4–6 hrs.)[3]	**Ultrashort acting (15–30 min.)[4]**
Amylobarbitone, Butobarbitone	Thiopentone, Thiamylal
Aprobarbital	Methohexital

Mainly used as anticonvulsants[1], for induction of sleep[2], in insomnia to maintain sleep[3], as general anesthetics[4].

As far as the toxicity of barbiturates is concerned, above classification does not hold true as duration of CNS depression after an acute overdose is comparable for all, except phenobarbital and primidone, which exert toxicity features for prolonged duration because of their long elimination $t_{1/2}$.

Mechanism of toxicity

All barbiturates cause generalized neuronal depression in the brain via enhanced GABA mediated inhibition of neurotransmission. Marked hypotension in overdose is caused by vasomotor depression and direct depression of cardiac contractility. Ultrashort acting barbiturates have high lipid solubility, potency and more toxicity than long acting ones, because they can more easily and rapidly penetrate the blood brain barrier and quickly redistribute to other tissues, so their duration of action is much shorter in contrast to long acting ones.

Toxic dose

The toxicity of barbiturates varies widely and depends on the dose, polarity of the compound, route of administration, sensitivity of the patient (abuser/chronic user) and concomitant administration of other CNS depressants. In general, toxicity occurs when dose exceeds 5–10 times the therapeutic hypnotic dose.

Long acting barbiturates

Long acting barbiturates may produce toxicity at 8 mg/kg dose. However, a dose of upto 1000 mg of phenobarbital has been tolerated by the addicts. Plasma levels of more than 80 μg/ml of primidone are associated with some degree of coma. Minimum toxic levels for mephobarbital and phenobarbital are >30 mg/L each.

Short acting barbiturates

Fatal dose of short acting barbiturates in non-addicted adults is 3–6 g. The toxic dose in children is 5–8 mg/kg. Fatalities are reported with the ingestion of as low as 2 g of secobarbital. Blood concentrations vary from 5 to 52 μg/ml. Coma may occur when levels reach 18 μg/ml. Levels of 24 μg/ml or greater may result in severe intoxication leading to respiratory depression and hypotension. The minimum toxic levels of methohexital and thiopental are >5 mg/L each and for pentobarbitone, secobarbitone, amobarbital, aprobarbital, butabarbital are >10 mg/L each. Fatalities are reported with the ingestion of 2–10 g of pentobarbital. Coma may be seen at plasma levels of 28 μg/ml.

Clinical features

Long acting

- Manifestations of toxicity start at 1–2 hrs. of exposure.
- In mild/moderate doses nystagmus, dysarthria, ataxia, drowsiness, bullae and crystaluria (primidone) are noted.
- In massive overdose features like coma, respiratory depression, aspiration, hypotension, hypothermia and acute renal failure are seen.
- Toxicity is enhanced with concomitant use of other CNS depressants.

Short acting

- CNS and respiratory depression, bullous skin lesions and aspiration pneumonia may be noted.
- Hypothermia is seen in mild to moderate poisoning.
- Renal failure, muscle necrosis, hypotension, hypoglycemia occur in severe poisoning.
- Toxicity is enhanced with concomitant use of other CNS depressants.

Diagnosis

Diagnosis is based on history of exposure and presenting clinical features. Barbiturate poisoning should be suspected in epileptic patients presenting with stupor or coma. Skin bullae may be seen in barbiturate poisoning, however, it is not the characteristic feature of poisoning. Rule out other causes of bullae and coma. A few drugs (tricyclics and benzodiazepines) and chemicals may produce bullae. Coma may be seen with general CNS depressants, sympatholytic agents, in cellular hypoxia and by certain other toxins.

Laboratory/Monitoring

- Blood levels of barbiturates are unreliable in predicting the duration and severity of overdose and are closely related to the concentrations in the brain rather than plasma.
- Plasma levels of 3.5 mg/dl and 10mg/L for short and long acting barbiturates respectively, indicate severe toxicity. However, the quantitative assays just measure barbiturate moiety and do not differentiate between various barbiturates.
- Monitor electrolytes, glucose, BUN, creatinine, arterial blood gases or pulse oximetry and chest X-ray.

Management

Pre-hospital

- Induce emesis with syrup of ipecac immediately within few minutes of ingestion.
- Administer activated charcoal.

Hospital

- Secure the airway and provide ventilatory support if required.
- Correct hypotension with IV fluids and vasopressors.
- Perform gastric lavage preferably within 1 hr. of ingestion.
- Treat withdrawal symptoms with IV benzodiazepine/barbiturate as needed.
- Multiple dose activated charcoal may enhance elimination.
- Perform forced alkaline diuresis with IV furosemide.
- Forced alkaline diuresis is of little value in short acting barbiturate poisoning.
- Charcoal hemoperfusion/hemodialysis is recommended in severe hypotension and is highly effective, however it is less efficacious in poisoning by short acting barbiturates.
- Analeptics like metrazol and bemegride are contraindicated because of their narrow margin of safety and precipitation of convulsions

even in comatose patients. Chances of mortality may increase. Doxapram may be used initially before providing respiratory support.

Antihistamines

Antihistamines antagonize the histamine (tissue amine) mediated effects in the body. The response of histamine is mediated via 3 distinct histamine receptors H_1, H_2 and H_3. H_1 receptors are present in the smooth muscles of bronchi, blood vessels, heart, CNS, autonomic ganglia and afferent nerve fibres and mediate the allergic and inflammatory response. H_2 receptors are present on gastric parietal cells, vascular smooth muscles, heart, CNS and T lymphocytes. They are mainly responsible for gastric acid secretion. H_3 receptors are present presynaptically on nerve terminals in the brain and periphery.They mediate the feedback control of histamine synthesis and release. The chemical classification of antihistamines is given in Table 2.

Table 2.   Classification of antihistamines

H_1 Antihistamines
First generation

Ethanolamines	Carbinoxamine maleate, clemastine fumarate, diphenhydramine hydrochloride, diphenylpyraline, dimenhydrinate, doxylamine.
Ethylenediamines	Pyrilamine maleate, tripelennamine hydrochloride, tripelennamine citrate, antazoline, chlorothen, clemizole, mepyramine.
Alkylamines	Pheniramine maleate, chlorpheniramine (chlorphenamine) maleate, brompheniramine maleate, dimethindene, triprolidine.
Piperazines	Hydroxyzine hydrochloride, hydroxyzine pamoate, cyclizine hydrochloride, cyclizine lactate, chlorcyclizine, meclizine hydrochloride, dimethothiazine, methdilazine, trimeprazine.
Phenothiazines	Promethazine hydrochloride, chlorpromazine.
Piperidines	Bamipine, cyproheptadine, pizotifen.

Second generation

Pyridines	Acrivastine.
Piperazines	Cetrizine hydrochloride.
Piperidines	Astemizole, terfenadine, loratadine, levocabastine hydrochloride.
Miscellaneous	Ebastine, azelastine, emedastine, ketotifen, mizolastine, oxatomide, fexofenadine.

H_2 Antihistamines

Imidazole derivatives	Cimetidine.
Furan derivatives	Ranitidine.
Thiazole derivatives	Famotidine, nizetidine.
Miscellaneous	Roxatadine acetate, zolentidine.
H_3 Antihistamines	Thioperamide, clobenpropit.

H_1 antihistamines (particularly of first generation) are the ingredients of several common cold, cough and sleep medications. They are available as tablets, capsules, syrups, suspensions, injectables etc. They are used in the treatment of allergic disorders, anaphylactic shock, motion sickness, vestibular disease (Meniere's disease), preanaesthetic medication, insect bites, common cold, Parkinson's disease, vomiting, asthma, insomnia etc.

H_2 antihistamines are used in the treatment of duodenal ulcers, gastric ulcers, Zollinger-Ellison syndrome, systemic mastocytosis and basophilic leukemia, reflux esophagitis, stress ulcers, iatrogenic ulcers, hiatus hernia, short bowel (anastomosis) syndrome, preanaesthetic medication in emergency operations to reduce the danger of aspiration of acidic gastric contents. They are also being used to treat allergic reactions.

Mechanism of toxicity
H_1 Antihistamines competitively antagonize the histamine mediated actions at H_1 receptor sites. The first generation H_1 antihistamines possess anticholinergic and cardiac membrane stabilizing properties. The anticholinergic and sedative properties are less marked with second generation H_1 antihistamines. Terfenadine, astemizole and loratadine are devoid of their effects on muscarinic receptors. At relatively large doses, diphenhydramine hydrochloride and promethazine hydrochloride possess local anaesthetic effects. First generation antihistamines also have antiserotonergic (cyproheptadine, indoramin) and α-adrenergic receptor blocking properties (indoramin, chlorpromazine).

H_2 antihistamines competitively block the interaction of histamine on H_2 receptors and inhibit the secretion of HCl from gastric parietal cells. They also inhibit the acid secretion elicited by gastrin as well as to a lesser extent by muscarinic agonists.

Toxic dose

First generation H_1 antihistamines
The ratio of therapeutic/toxic dose of H_1 antihistamines is high. In general, H_1 antihistamines induce toxicity at 3–5 times the therapeutic dose. Accidental poisoning is more likely in children than adults. Children are more susceptible to toxicity. Toxic dose of cyclizine is 5 mg/kg in adults and children. Its lethal dose is 80 mg/kg. Severe toxicity is observed at 5 g (80 mg/kg) of dimenhydrinate. Toxic dose of doxylamine succinate in children is >1.8 mg/kg. Fatality has been reported in a 3 year old child at the dose of 1000 mg. Hydroxizine causes toxic features at the dose of 1–2 g in adults.

Second generation H_1 antihistamines
Little information is available regarding their toxic dose. Toxicity occurs with astemizole at therapeutic drug levels because of its interaction with

drugs which inhibit cytochrome P-450 enzyme (e.g. erythromycin, ketoconazole etc.). Usually large doses of other agents produce toxicity.

H_2 Antihistamines

Cimetidine causes mild to moderate toxicity upto the acute dose of 20 g. Death has been reported with the ingestion of 24 g in an adult female. Experience with overdose of nizatidine is lacking at the moment. However, very high doses are relatively non toxic in animals.

Clinical features

First generation H_1 antihistamines

- Toxicity symptoms start within half an hour to 2 hrs. post ingestion.
- Mild CNS and psychomotor excitation (predominant in young children) to CNS depression, hyperthermia, convulsions (more likely with pheniramine), coma and death may occur.
- Anticholinergic toxicities include fixed and dilated pupils, blurred vision, diplopia, dryness of mouth and nose, tightness in the chest, nausea and constipation or diarrhea.
- Tinnitus and acute labyrinthytis is also reported. Adynamic ileus is the most troublesome GI toxic effect.
- Dystonic reactions, dyskinesia, choreoathetosis are seen in cyproheptadine overdose.
- CNS toxicity is also predominant in cyproheptadine overdose.
- Myocardial depression and QRS widening with syncope has been reported in severe intoxication with diphenhydramine hydrochloride.
- Rhabdomyolysis has been seen in overdose of doxylamine succinate.
- Hyperpyrexia, status epilepticus, cardiac arrhythmias and coma are observed in severe toxicity of dimenhydrinate.

Second generation H_1 antihistamines

- Dizziness, syncope, QT prolongation, *torsade de pointes* are seen in mild toxicity of astemizole and terfenadine.
- Toxicity, particularly cardiac conduction abnormalities are further worsened in severe intoxication and in patients taking erythromycin, ketoconazole or other cytochrome P-450 inhibitors.

H_2 antihistamines

- Cardiotoxicity (bradycardia, hypotension, sinus arrest) is reported with IV overdose of various H_2 antihistamines.
- CNS symptoms are rare and include from drowsiness and lethargy to agitation, hallucinations, seizures etc. Risk of CNS toxicity is increased in geriatric population and in pathologic states (hepatic and renal disease).

- Cimetidine rarely causes reversible bone marrow depression, hepatitis and anaphylaxis.
- Other H_2 antihistamines which differ from cimetidine in their chemical structure have similar adverse effects, however they are less likely to inhibit cytochrome P-450.
- Overdose with nizatidine may cause cholinergic toxicity (lacrimation, salivation, emesis, miosis and diarrhea).

Diagnosis

Diagnosis of first generation H_1 antihistamines is based on history of exposure and typical anticholinergic symptoms. Rule out the possibility of ingestion of cyclic antidepressants, antiparkinsonian agents, antipsychotics, antispasmodics, belladonna alkaloids, mydriatics, skeletal muscle relaxants, mushrooms and other toxic plants that cause sedation and anticholinergic effects. Second generation H_1 antihistamines have negligible affinity for cholinergic, α-adrenergic, serotonergic and dopamine receptors and consequently do not inhibit these receptors. The widely used antihistamines may be detected in urine samples.

Laboratory/Monitoring

H_1 Antihistamines

- Blood levels are not usually available and clinically useful.
- Monitor electrolytes, glucose, arterial blood gases, ECG (diphenhydramine, terfenadine, astemizole, ebastine).
- Monitoring of myoglobin in urine will rule out diphenhydramine and doxylamine intoxication.

H_2 Antihistamines

- Blood levels are not usually available and clinically useful.
- Monitor CBC, electrolytes, urine, cardiac functions, CNS, endocrine, liver and renal functions in overdose.

Management

Pre-hospital

- Administer activated charcoal.
- Induce emesis with syrup of ipecac immediately (within first few minutes of ingestion).

Hospital

- Administer activated charcoal and a cathartic. Repeat dose activated charcoal is not effective.

- Perform gastric lavage preferably within 1 hr. of ingestion. However, it may be done after an hour also.
- Do not use antipyretics (salicylates) in hyperthermia. Physical cooling is recommended.
- Treat agitation and seizures with anticonvulsants. Control recurrent seizures with phenytoin/phenobarbital.
- Treat sinus tachycardia with IV fluids.
- Control agitation induced tachycardia initially with a BDZ before giving antiarrhythmics.
- Physostigmine is used to treat severe central and peripheral anticholinergic symptoms (narrow QRS complex, refractory supraventricular tachycardia with either haemodynamic instability or ischaemic chest pain) not responding to other agents as antihistamines carry the risk of development of seizures in overdose.
- Treat *Torsade de pointes* with IV magnesium sulphate.
- Treat myocardial depression and QRS interval prolongation with IV sodium bicarbonate.
- Manage hypotension with IV fluids and vasopressors. Avoid epinephrine.
- Consider isoproterenol, cardioversion and overdrive pacing in life threatening arrhythmias (*torsade de pointes* complicated by hypotension, myocardial ischaemia or congestive cardiac failure).
- Forced diuresis is not effective.
- Role of hemodialysis, hemoperfusion, peritoneal dialysis and exchange transfusion is questionable.
- Hemodialysis and hemoperfusion have been shown to be effective in cimetidine and ranitidine overdose only experimentally.
- Monitor cardiac status for 18-24 hrs. post ingestion of terfenadine and astemizole.
- There is no specific antidote.

Opioids

Opioids are the natural, semisynthetic or synthetic compounds having opium (Afim) or morphine like actions. Opium is a dark brown resinous material obtained from the dried juice of unripe poppy capsules (*Papaver somniferum*) after incision. Opioids are administered orally and parenterally and are available alone and in combination with salicylates. They are used as analgesics in severe pain, in acute left ventricular failure (cardiac asthma), preanaesthetic medication, balanced anaesthesia and neurolept analgesia and for the relief of anxiety and apprehension. They are also used for the relief of cough and diarrhea. Apart from clinical uses, they are also the drugs of abuse.

Mechanism of toxicity
The toxicity of a particular opioid depends on its nature and relative affinity

for interaction with different receptors. Opioids are thought to mediate their toxicity through interaction with 3 distinct opioid receptors such as μ, k and δ present in the CNS and intestine. However, the major involvement is of μ receptors (μ_2 subtype) leading particularly to their sedative, respiratory depressant and cardiovascular depressant effects and decreased GI motility. Respiratory and circulatory failure leads to death.

Toxic dose
The toxic doses vary depending on the compound involved, its potency and elimination $t_{1/2}$, rate and route of exposure, concomitant use of other CNS depressants as well as the environment in which it is administered. Circadian variations also contribute to individual's sensitivity to opioid overdose. Larger doses are required in addicts for toxic features to be evident. Concomitant administration of other CNS depressants decreases the latency and augments the toxic features. The adult lethal dose of morphine is 200–250 mg. The features of codeine intoxication are manifested at the dose of 2 mg/kg and death occurs with 500–1000 mg. The adult fatal dose of methadone is 50 mg. A rare case of fatal tramadol intoxication with peripheral blood concentration of 9.6 mg/L has been reported in an adult. Fatal fentanyl poisoning (100 mg/hr. fentanyl patches) has been reported in an elderly female following excessive transdermal application. Acute IV heroin intoxication has been shown to cause death in most cases within 1–3 hours.

Clinical features
- Classical features are CNS depression (lethargy), respiratory depression and miosis. The pupils may also be dilated if the patient is hypoxic. Other features are bradycardia, decrease in blood pressure, body temperature and pulse rate, decreased gastric motility or bowel sounds.
- Severe symptoms include profound respiratory and circulatory depression, cardiac arrest, rhabdomyolysis, renal failure and anoxic encephalopathy. Naloxone resistant non-cardiogenic pulmonary edema may be seen with heroin, codeine, methadone and morphine.
- Seizures are common with codeine, dextropropoxyphene, diphenoxylate, pethidine (meperidine) and dextromethorphan intoxication. Heroin also causes seizures. Seizure threshold is decreased in patients with renal impairment.
- Fulminant but reversible pulmonary edema is reported in heroin intoxication. Pneumonia may also occur.
- Cardiac arrhythmias are not common, however, may be seen within minutes after IV injection and within an hour after oral ingestion in dextropropoxyphene poisoning.
- Cardiac arrhythmias may be delayed in case of methadone. The same is true for slow release formulations also.
- Toxic symptoms are unpredictable with overdose of newly synthesized mixed opioid agonist-antagonists.

Diagnosis

Diagnosis is based on history of exposure and classical triad of opioid intoxication [pin point pupils, respiratory depression, CNS depression (coma)]. Rule out the intoxication with combination of NSAIDs particularly salicylates and paracetamol. Needle track marks are suggestive of IV drug use in addicts.

Laboratory/Monitoring

- There is no perfect correlation between specific drug levels and presenting clinical features.
- Levels of synthetic opioids are not routinely available.
- Monitor electrolytes, glucose, arterial blood gases and chest X-ray.
- Estimate stat serum paracetamol/salicylate levels (in combination formulations).
- Perform urinalysis.
- Monitor multisystem organ functions such as CNS, respiration and cardiac status.

Management

Pre-hospital

- Ipecac induced emesis is contraindicated, however, it can be done immediately within few minutes of exposure.
- Administer activated charcoal.

Hospital

- Secure the airway. Use ventilatory support if required.
- Administer activated charcoal and a cathartic (sorbitol or magnesium sulphate). Gastric lavage is not required if charcoal is administered promptly.
- Administer thiamine and glucose in patients showing altered consciousness.
- Treat non-cardiogenic pulmonary edema with naloxone and oxygen. Positive end expiratory pressure (PEEP) may be required for adequate oxygenation.
- Treat hypotension with IV fluids and vasopressors.
- Control seizures by correcting hypoxia and using anticonvulsants.
- There is no role of dialysis.
- Naloxone is the specific antidote.

Lithium

Lithium is a small, readily diffusible monovalent cation. It has mood stabilizing activity, narrow margin of safety and slow onset of action. It is available for oral administration only. It is used for the prophylaxis and treatment of manic depression, prophylaxis of bipolar manic depressive illness, recurrent unipolar depression, schizophrenia and schizoaffective disorders, impulse control disorders and aggression and in a variety of other clinical conditions like cancer chemotherapy induced myelosuppression (leucopenia, agranulocytosis), inappropriate ADH secretion syndrome, alcoholism etc.

Mechanism of toxicity
Lithium has chemical similarity to that of sodium, potassium and calcium. Its mean serum half life is 20.9 hrs. It is capable of displacing these electrolytes (sodium, potassium, magnesium and calcium) from intracellular and bone sites in this order. It stabilizes cell membranes by multiple mechanisms: (a) by inhibiting the release and enhancing the uptake of noradrenaline at nerve terminals. (b) by inhibiting hydro-osmotic effect of arginine vasopressin through reduction of receptor mediated synthesis of c-AMP, as a result of inhibition of adenylate cyclase (possible mechanism in nephrogenic diabetes incipidus and impairment of thyroid function). Apart from these, other mechanisms are also involved in lithium intoxication.

Toxic dose
The exact acute toxic dose of lithium is not established. Chronic lithium poisoning is more common and serious as compared with acute poisoning. Significant toxicity may not be observed after acute lithium intoxication till the levels are more than 4 mEq/L. The normal serum lithium levels range from 0.6 to 1.2 mEq/L. A case of acute lithium intoxication during pregnancy leading to fetal CNS depression and premature delivery has been reported. A case of acute lithium overdose (97 immediate release lithium carbonate tablets, 300 mg each orally and 80 tablets intravaginally) has been reported in a 48 year old female of bipolar disorder and a history of border line personality disorder. The symptoms developed were mild lethargy, decreased patellar reflexes, mild T-wave flattening in ECG and intense vaginal burning. In one more case, acute mixed ingestion of lithium carbonate (22.5 g) + thioridazine (1.25 g) in a 58 year old female did not cause fatality and serum lithium levels were as high as 8.2 mEq/L at 2.5 hrs. after ingestion without any CNS toxicity.

Clinical features

- Nausea, vomiting and diarrhea occur within an hour of acute intoxication.
- Neurological features may be delayed (several hours to days as lithium takes time to move into intracellular compartment). Mild to moderate features include lethargy, muscle weakness, ataxia, tremors, myoclonic jerks and extrapyramidal symptoms.
- Severe features are restlessness, convulsions, agitated delirium,

hyperthermia, neuromuscular irritability, polydypsia, polyuria, gastroenteritis, respiratory failure, ARDS and coma.
- Diabetes incipidus and hypothyroidism may develop.
- Cardiac abnormalities are T-wave inversion in ECG, myocarditis, bradycardia and sinus node arrest.
- WBC and neutrophil count is raised.
- Anticholinergic features are usually not seen.
- Recovery from lithium poisoning is very slow, patient may be confused or obtunded for a long time (several days to week).

Diagnosis

Those patients who have a history of psychiatric disorders are potential candidates to be suspected for lithium intoxication. The irreversible neurological sequalae are usually the cerebeller signs especially the ataxia and dysarthria after acute lithium intoxication. The diagnosis can be confirmed by estimating stat serum lithium levels (though it is not an accurate predictor of toxicity because of its continuous absorption from the GI tract) to give an idea of severity of poisoning. The peak serum levels may be several times higher than normal after acute intoxication, without noticeable signs of toxicity. In contrast, patients on chronic lithium therapy may show neurological symptoms at normal serum lithium levels or only marginally higher than normal. Low anion gap also aids in the diagnosis.

Laboratory/Monitoring

- Monitor stat serum lithium levels and then at regular intervals of 2–4 hrs. until symptoms are controlled. The peak serum lithium levels occur at 1–4 hrs. after ingestion of immediate release lithium carbonate tablets.
- With slow or extended release formulations, the peak effect may be delayed for more than 8 hrs. Sometimes multiple peaks may also be present.
- Regularly monitor ECG, hemodynamic parameters, electrolytes, glucose, BUN, creatinine etc.

Management

Pre-hospital

- Induce emesis with syrup of ipecac.

Hospital

- Treatment is supportive and symptomatic.
- Secure the airway. Use ventilatory support if required.

- Activated charcoal is not a good adsorbant of lithium ions, however, still try one dose if a coingestant is suspected.
- Perform gastric lavage as early as possible (preferably within 2 hrs.). Most reports suggest that the gastric lavage may be done within first 24–48 hrs. post ingestion.
- Perform whole bowel irrigation in massive overdose or slow release formulations using balanced electrolyte solution containing polyethylene glycol (PEG) and continue till rectal effluent is as clear as the PEG being administered.
- Sodium polystyrene sulphonate resin administration has been shown to be effective experimentally and clinically, its routine use is not recommended, as lower limits of its effective dosing and extent of potassium lowering effect is questionable.
- Maintain fluid, electrolyte balance and normothermia. Hydration (normal saline) is shown to enhance renal lithium elimination. The concentration of normal saline may be reduced to half of the original, once initial hydration is completed.
- Rehydrate severely dehydrated patients following lithium intoxication.
- Forced diuresis with thiazide (hydrochlorthiazide) and high ceiling diuretics (like furosemide) is not effective. Use furosemide in volume overloaded patients. IV mannitol and IV sodium bicarbonate slightly increase lithium excretion.
- IV aminophylline may be useful in decreasing absorption and enhancing lithium excretion, however, extensive studies are lacking and its risks outweigh possible benefits.
- Treat refractory cardiac arrhythmias with injectable magnesium sulphate and sodium bicarbonate.
- Intermittent hemodialysis is a well documented and effective means of enhancing lithium elimination and is strongly recommended in severely intoxicated patients, (absolute level > 4 mEq/L at 6 hrs. post ingestion and continue till lithium level is <0.5 mEq/L). This process, however, carries the risk of post dialysis rebound elevation in lithium concentration (peak at 4–13 hrs.), collapse and recurrent aggravation of hemodynamic instability.
- Peritoneal dialysis may be used if hemodialysis is unavailable.
- Continuous renal replacement therapy (continuous arteriovenous and venovenous diafiltration) or low dose dopamine have been documented to enhance lithium elimination in case of acute on chronic lithium intoxication.
- Monitor for persistant neurological ('coma vigil' characterized by catatonia and the eyes looking in the state of ever looking and vigilant) and renal deterioration. Consult a neurologist and/nephrologist as the case may be.
- There is no specific antidote.

Tricyclic antidepressants

Antidepressants refer to the drugs used to treat depression of varied clinical etiology. They can be classified into different groups as tricyclic antidepressants (TCAs), monoamine oxidase (MAO) inhibitors, selective serotonin reuptake inhibitors (SSRIs) and miscellaneous agents (Table 3).

Table 3. Major groups of antidepressants

Tricyclic antidepressants	MAO inhibitors
Imipramine, desipramine, amitriptyline, nortriptyline, protriptyline, clomipramine, doxepin, trimipramine, amoxepine, butriptyline, amineptine, dothiepin, nitroxazepine.	Non-selective: Phenelzine, nialamide, isocarboxazid, tranylcypromine. Selective MAO-A: Clorgiline. Selective MAO-B: Moclobemide, selegiline.
Selective serotonin reuptake inhibitors (SSRIs)	**Miscellaneous agents**
Fluoxetine, fluvoxamine, paroxetine, sertraline, venlafaxine.	Tianeptine, trazodone, mianserin, bupropion, nefazodone.

Presently TCAs and SSRIs are considered to be the first line drugs for the treatment of mild to moderate depression. SSRIs are however, the treatment of choice owing to their superior safety profile. They are not indicated in severe depression where electroconvulsive therapy is used. All antidepressants have almost equal efficacy and latency after which their therapeutic effects become evident. Apart from major and minor depressive disorders they are indicated in a variety of medical and psychiatric conditions. Some indications are however, not approved by US FDA and are considered to be the "off label" indications. The indications of antidepressants include major depression, recurrent depression, depressive phase of bipolar disorders, prophylaxis of mania-depressive disorders, obsessive compulsive disorders (clomipramine), panic disorders, post traumatic stress disorders, bulimia nervosa (fluoxetine), premenstrual tension (fluoxetine recently approved by FDA), prophylaxis of generalized anxiety disorders*, chronic pain (neuropathy, cancer pain), fibromyalgias, nocturnal enuresis (imipramine), sleep apnea syndrome*, chronic urticaria*, attention deficit hyperkinetic disorders etc.

Mechanism of toxicity

Inhibition of catecholamines (norepinephrine, dopamine, serotonin) reuptake in various nerve terminals contributes to their deleterious effects on heart. They also competitively block muscarinic, cholinergic, α-adrenergic, 5-HT, histamine (H_1 and H_2) and GABA receptors. Direct cardiac membrane depression leading to delayed depolarization and cardiac conduction abnormalities is one of the important mechanisms of their toxicity in overdose.

---

*off-label indications.

Toxic dose

10–20 mg/kg orally of most antidepressants causes moderate to severe toxicity in adults. The toxic and fatal doses in children are 3.5 mg/kg and 15 mg/kg respectively. Fatalities have been reported in children with as little as 250 mg of imipramine. Complete revival has been possible with acute overdose of upto 1.25 g of nortryptyline. Ingestion of 2.95 g of desipramine in an adult-female produced severe toxicity. Severe toxicity has been reported with 100 mg of desipramine in children. Topical application of 1.32 g of doxepin cream in a 5 year old child caused CNS depression, hypotension and tachycardia. Fatalities have been reported with 3–5 g of amoxepine in adults and with as little as 250 mg in children.

Clinical features

- Toxic effects of TCAs are usually manifested within 6 hrs. of acute overdose ingestion.
- Characteristic symptoms include QRS widening, cardiac conduction defects, arrhythmias, hypotension, psychological complications, hyperthermia, seizures and coma.
- Rhabdomyolysis, acute renal failure, adult respiratory distress syndrome (ARDS), acid base imbalance (acidosis) may complicate severe overdose.
- Seizures, respiratory arrest and coma have been reported with oral ingestion of as little as 100 mg imipramine in a 13 year old male child.
- Seizures, respiratory arrest, cardiac arrhythmias and circulatory collapse have been noted in severe intoxication with desipramine.
- Nortriptyline overdose produces relatively less hypotension than imipramine.
- Cardiac failure and pulmonary edema are reported in amoxepine overdose.

Diagnosis

Diagnosis should be suspected in patients having a history of depression and those showing characteristic cardiac and CNS toxicity features.

Laboratory/Monitoring

- Levels of TCAs are not useful in the initial assessment as they do not predict the clinical symptoms.
- Monitor ECG (QRS interval prolongation), electrolytes, bicarbonates, pH, renal and liver function tests, CPK, arterial blood gases, urinalysis, chest X-ray in patients suspected of significant toxicity and patients presenting with pulmonary symptoms.
- Perform qualitative tests.
- Serum/plasma levels of TCAs can be detected by immunoassays.

- HPLC and GC-MS have been employed to detect TCAs in hairs.
- Monitor serum paracetamol and aspirin levels to detect occult ingestion.

Management

Pre-hospital

- Do not induce emesis with syrup of ipecac because of risk of abrupt development of coma or seizures.
- Prevent aspiration in case of spontaneous emesis.
- Administer activated charcoal preferably within 1 hr. of ingestion.
- Protect airway in patients who are at risk of sudden onset of seizures or have undergone mental status deterioration.

Hospital

- Treatment is supportive and symptomatic.
- Perform early gastric lavage (within 1–1.5 hrs. post ingestion). However, late gastric lavage and charcoal may also be useful.
- Treat arrhythmias (QRS widening) with IV sodium bicarbonate. If arrhythmias do not respond to sodium bicarbonate, lidocaine may be given. Continuous sodium bicarbonate infusion is not recommended.
- Treat seizures with anticonvulsants, control recurrent seizures with phenytoin/phenobarbital or other class I_A antiarrhythmics.
- Correct hypotension with IV fluids and vasopressors if required.
- Maintain respiration.
- Dialysis and diuresis are not effective.
- Do not administer flumazenil, procainamide, quinidine, disopyramide.
- There is no specific antidote.

2. Pesticides

Organophosphates

Organophosphates (OPs) are lipophilic compounds formulated in petroleum distillates as emulsifiable concentrates or suspensions. Wettable powders, dusts and granules are also available. Some products are formulated as impregnated resins, fogging formulations or smokes. They are used extensively as insecticides, miticides and amphicides in agriculture and horticulture contributing maximum to the incidence and mortality due to acute poisonings. Certain rapid acting OPs have been developed as "nerve gases" for chemical warfare. Various petroleum distillates in which they are formulated may also cause toxic or irritant effects.

Common formulations

Acephate: Acatin, Acehero, Acekill, Acemil, Acet, Acetop, Acifete, Agrophate, Amithene, Artin, Asataf, Delthene, Dhanraj, Hilphate, Hythane, Lancer, Orthene Pace, Specthane, Starthene Tamaron gold, Tarpedo 75 WP, Tremor, Volace.

Azinphos methyl: Gusathion M, Guthion.

Chlorfenvinphos: Birlane, Chlorofenvinphos.

Chlorpyriphos: Agro-Chlore, Agrophos 20, Blaze, Chlorguard, Chlorofos 20, Classic Coroban 20, Corocin, Cyphos, Dhanwan 20, Doomer, Durmet 20 EC, Dursban, Force, Gilphos, Hexaban, Hilban, Hyban 20, Nuklor 20 EC, Pyrivol, Radar, Robust, Ruban 20, Scoui, Specphos 20, Starban, Strike, Sulban Tafaban, Tagaban 20 EC, Tarkash.

Diazinon: Agrozinon, Basudin, Bazanon, Suzinon, Zionosul-20.

Dichlorvos: Agro-DDVP, Agro 76 EC, Agrovan, Amidos, Bangvas, Dicotop, Ddoom, Divap, Divap 100, Divisol, Hilfol, Luvon, Mafu fogger, Marvex, Nuvan, Nuvasul 76, Paradeep, Savious, Specvos, Suchlor, Super, Vantaf, Vapona, Vapox, Vegfru.

Dimethoate: Agrodimet 30, Agromet 30 EC, Bangoor 30 EC, Champ, Cropgor 30, Diadhan, Dimethoate, Dimetox, Dimex, Entogor, Hexagor, Hilthoate, Hygro 30, Klex dimethoate, Milgor, Nugor, Paragor, Paragor 30, Parrydimate, Primer, Ramgor, Rogor, Specgor, Sulgor, Tafgor, Tagor, Tara 909, Teeka, Tophoate, Vikagor.

Edifenphos: Hinosan.

Ethion: Acarin, Dhan-unit, Ethion, Ethiosul 50, Force, Fosmite, Indothion, Lazer, Mit 505, Miticil, Phosmil, RP-Thion EC, RP-Thion 50 EC, Rafethion, Tafethion, Vegfru Fosmite, Volthion.

Fenitrothion: Agrothion, Fenicol, Fentrosul 50, Folithion, Hexafen, Sumithion, Tik-20, Vikathion.

Fenthion: Agrocidin, Baytex, Fenthiosul, Lebaycid.

Formothion: Anthio.

Isofenphos: Oftanol 500 EC.

Malathion: Agromal, Cythion, Dhanuka Malathion, Hilmala, Malamar Malatop, Finit, Kathion, Licel, Maladan, Malazene, Malataf, Maltox, Luthion Specmal, Sulmathion Vegfru malatox.

Methyl Parathion: Agro-Para, Agrotex, Devithion Dhanumar, Folidol-M, Luthion, Metacid, Metapar, Milion, Parahit, Paramar M, Parataf, Paratox, Tagpar.

Methamidophos: Monitor, Nitofol, Tamaron 600 SL.

Monocrotophos: Agromonark, Atom, Azodrin, Balwan, Bilphos, Corophos, Croton, Hilcron, Hycrophos, Kadett, Luphos, Macrophos Milphos, Moncar, Monochem, Monocil, Monocin, Monocron, Monophos, Monosect, Monostar, Monodhan, Monovol, Nuvacron, Parryphos, Phoskill, Specron, Sufos, Topcil.

Oxydemeton methyl: Dhanusystox, Hexasystox, Knock Out, Metasystox, Mode Metasystemox.

Omethoate: Folimat 500 SL, LE-MAT.

Phorate: Agro-Phorate, Agro-Phorate Phoratox, Dhan 100, Dragnet, Foratox, Forcin, Granutox, Grenade, Helmet, Hilphorate, Luphate, Milate, Specphor, Starphor, Thinmet, Umet, Volphor, Warrant.

Phosalone: Voltas, Zolone.

Phosphamidon: Agromidon 85 WSC, Aimphon, Bangdon 85 WSC, Cildon, Dimecron, Entecron 85, Hawk, Hydan, Phamidon, Phamodon, Phosul, Rilon, Specmidon, Sudon, Sumidon, Topcron, Umeson, Vimidon.

Phoxim: Baythion, Volaton 2,5-GR.

Prothiofos: Tokuthion 450 EC.

Quinalphos: Agroquin, Agroquinol, Basquin, Bayrusil, Chemlux, Dhanulux, Ekalux, Ekatop, Flash, Hilquin, Hyquin, Kinalux, Knock, Krush, Quick, Quinal, Quinguard, Quinaltaf, Quinatox, Shakti, Smash, Starlux, Suquin, Tagquin, Vazra, Volquin.

Sulprofos: Bolstar 720 EC, Helothion.

Temephos: Abate.

Trizophos: Hostathion, Trelka.

Methamidophos + Cyfluthrin: Baythroid TM 525 EC, Magnum 525 SL.

Methamidophos + Triflumuron: Tamaron Combi 330 EC.

Chlorpyriphos +Cypermethrin: Nurelle D 505.

Mechanism of toxicity

Exposure to organophosphates results in inhibition of the enzymes acetyl-cholinesterase (AChE) and plasma cholinesterase. The enzyme AChE gets phosphorylated and the resultant phosphorylated enzyme is extremely stable requiring several hours to days for reactivation. There is accumulation of acetylcholine at the nerve endings, the excess of which initially stimulates and subsequently paralyzes cholinergic synaptic transmission in the CNS, somatic nerves, autonomic ganglia, parasympathetic nerve endings and some sympathetic nerve endings.

Some highly lipophilic OPs like disulfoton, fenthion etc. are stored in fat tissues which may lead to delayed and persistent toxicity for several days after exposure.

Toxic dose

Acute toxicity of organophosphates is variable depending on absorption kinetics and whether or not metabolic activation is required. Sudden absorption of a less toxic compound may have a more severe effect. Compounds used in agriculture are most toxic, those used in animal husbandry have intermediate toxicity and the ones used for household pest control and for human ectoparasites are least toxic. On the basis of oral LD_{50} values in rat the toxicity of various compounds has been classified as high, moderate and low (Table 1).

Table 1. Classification of organophosphates

Mild toxicity	Moderate toxicity	Severe toxicity
Iodofenphos	Acephate	Chlorfenvinphos
Malathion	Chlorpyriphos	Demeton
Primiphos-methyl	Diazinon	Dicrotophos
Temephos	Dichlofenthion	Isofenphos
	Dichlorvos	Monocrotophos
	Dimethoate	Parathion
	Edifenphos	Phorate
	Ethion	Phosphamidon
	Fenitrothion	
	Fenthion	
	Formothion	
	Oxydemeton methyl	
	Phosalone	
	Profenophos	
	Propetamphos	
	Quinalphos	
	Triazophos	

Clinical features

- Muscarinic effects in moderate to severe poisoning include miosis, salivation, lacrimation, urination, defecation, gastrointestinal distress, emesis, bronchorrhea, bronchoconstriction, diaphoresis, bradycardia and hypotension.
- Bronchorrhea and bronchoconstriction may lead to compromised pulmonary functions including non-cardiogenic pulmonary edema along with chemical pneumonitis due to aspiration of hydrocarbon vehicle.
- Nicotinic effects include muscle fasciculations, cramps, hypertension, tachycardia, pupillary dilatation, weakness that can progress to areflexia and paralysis.
- Central nervous system effects in mild to moderate poisoning are headache, giddiness, anxiety, restlessness/drowsiness, confusion, tremors, slurred speech and generalized weakness.
- Delirium, psychosis, seizures, coma and cardiorespiratory depression are noted in severe cases.
- Delayed or permanent peripheral neuropathy may be developed, after 6-21 days of exposure, by some agents.
- Intermediate syndrome characterized by the development of proximal weakness and paralysis within 12 hrs. to 7 days of exposure has been observed. Signs of paralysis include inability to lift neck or sit up, slow eye movement, facial and limb weakness, difficulty in swallowing, areflexia and respiratory paralysis which may cause death.
- Mild inhalation exposure to vapours rapidly produces mucous membrane and upper airway irritation and bronchospasm followed by systemic symptoms if exposed to significant concentrations.
- Dermal exposure causes burning sensation, urticaria and angioedema.

Diagnosis

It involves history of exposure, characteristic muscarinic, nicotinic and CNS manifestations, breath odour of petroleum distillate and garlic. Qualitative test of lavage sample and determination of plasma and red blood cell cholinesterase activity also aid in the diagnosis.

Laboratory/Monitoring

- Depression of 25% or more in the red blood cell acetyl cholinesterase (AChE) activity from baseline indicates exposure. Plasma pseudocholinesterase, though a sensitive indicator, is not as reliable as AChE activity.
- Monitor electrolytes, glucose, BUN, creatinine, liver transaminases, arterial blood gases, serum pancreatic isoamylase, chest X-ray and ECG.
- Urine assay for alkyl phosphate and phenolic organophosphate metabolites may be a sensitive indicator of exposure.

Management

Pre-hospital

- Remove the patient from the source of exposure to fresh air.
- Remove contaminated clothing and discard leather items if any.
- Give artificial respiration if the patient is unable to breath, avoiding mouth to mouth breathing.
- Do not induce vomiting and lay patient on side to prevent aspiration of vomitus.
- In case of seizures, put a spoon in patient's mouth to prevent injury to tongue.
- Wash affected skin including hair and nails with copious amounts of soap and water and irrigate eyes with tepid water.
- Avoid contact with contaminated clothing and vomitus and wear rubber gloves while washing patient's skin or hair.
- Shift the patient to hospital and carry the container alongwith to aid diagnosis.

Hospital

- Ensure a clear airway by nasopharyngeal suction of vomitus and secretions.
- Provide oxygenation and ventilatory support as required.
- Perform gastric lavage cautiously protecting the airway in alert patients and using cuffed endotracheal tube in unconscious patients.
- Replace fluid loss by IV fluids.
- Administer activated charcoal as a slurry.
- Give cathartics for gut decontamination. Do not administer oil based cathartics like castor oil and liquid paraffin.
- Control seizures with anticonvulsants.
- Treat recurrent seizures with phenobarbital.
- Avoid using drugs like morphine, theophylline, succinylcholine and phenothiazines.
- Atropine and pralidoxime are the specific antidotes.

Organochlorines

Organochlorine compounds are widely used as pesticides in agriculture and as environmental pesticide control products. Commercial preparations are commonly dissolved in petroleum distillates which form emulsions when added to water. The γ-isomer of benzene hexachloride called lindane is used clinically as an ectoparasiticide. Organochlorines are of toxicological concern and some like dichloro diphenyl trichloroethane (DDT) and chlordane have been banned for commercial use as they persist in environment and accumulate in biological systems. Based on their chemical structure they are categorised into DDT and analogs, γ-benzene hexachloride and cyclodienes (aldrin, chlordane, endosulfan, heptachlor, toxaphene and related compounds).

Common formulations
Aldrin: Agroaldrin, Alcrop, Alditon, Aldrin, Mildrin 30 EC, Tarmahit 30.

Benzene hexachloride: Agrobenz D-10, Agro BHC, Hilbleach 50 WP, Kargo BHC, Premodole 10 EC, Solchlor, Sulbenz 50, Sudarsan, Sunbrand.

Chlordane: Agrodane 20 EC, Chlorodane, Mitox 20 EC, Sudarshan 20 EC, Termex, Vegfru Chlorotox.

DDT: DDT Sudarsan, Didinex 25 EC, Ramdit, Sun brand, Soltax, Suldit 50, Taforol.

Endosulfan: Thiodan, Endocol, Endosul, Endostar, Dawn, Hysulfan, Top Sulfan, Endocin, Parry Sulfan, Endodhan, Endonil, Endosol, Thiokill, Lusulfan, Agrosulfan, Hildan, Tagsulfan, Hexasulfan, Endotaf, Speed, Devigor.

Heptachlor: Agrochlor-D5, Heptar, Heptaf-50, Heptachlor, JOEC Heptachlor, Vegfru Heptex.

Lindane (gamma benzene hexachloride): Agrodane, Agrodono, Emscab., GAB, Gamaric, Gamascab, Higama, Lindex, Linsuline, Lindane 20, Lintox, Lindstar, Lintaf, Rasayan Lindane, Scabex, Scaboma, Scarab, Ultrascab.

Paradichloro benzene: Para DCB, Baansaka air freshner.

Mechanism of toxicity
Organochlorines affect the CNS nerve cells primarily interfering with the normal flux of sodium and potassium ions across the axon membrane resulting in behavioural changes, involuntary muscle activity and depression of the respiratory centre.

They are absorbed via inhalation, orally and transdermally. Presence of lipids enhances oral absorption which is generally efficient. However, the dermal absorption varies from compound to compound, while DDT has a poor skin absorption, dieldrin and lindane are efficiently absorbed through dermal route.

Toxic dose
The acute toxic doses of these compounds are highly variable. Aldrin, dieldrin, endrin are highly toxic organochlorines. While chlordane, DDT, hepatachlor, kepone, lindane, mirex and toxaphene are moderately toxic; methoxychlor, hexachlorobenzene and perthane have low toxicity. The estimated adult lethal oral dose of aldrin and chlordane is 3-7 g and of dieldrin is 2-5 g. A dose of 10-30 g of lindane is considered lethal in an adult while 1 g can produce seizures in a child.

Clinical features

- DDT and analogs cause nausea, vomiting, headache, dizziness, hyperesthesia, paresthesia (face and extremities), muscle incoordination, tremors, confusion, agitation, and ataxia.
- In severe poisoning, myoclonic jerking movements, opsoclonus, generalized tonic-clonic convulsions followed by coma, respiratory depression and death have been observed.
- Benzene hexachloride causes nausea, vomiting, diarrhea, seizures, headache, dizziness, numbness of hands and arms, ataxia, CNS depression and coma.
- Cyclodienes cause sudden onset of convulsions.
- Delayed and recurrent seizures are common with chlordane and aldrin.
- Aspiration of formulations containing petroleum distillates may result in pneumonitis.
- Fever secondary to central mechanisms, increased muscle activity and or aspiration pneumonitis is common with all the classes of organochlorines.
- Signs of hepatic or renal injury may develop.
- Inhalation of hexachlorobenzene may cause irritation of respiratory membranes.
- Extensive dermal contact causes irritation.

Diagnosis

It is mainly based on the history of exposure and clinical presentation.

Laboratory/Monitoring

- Monitor electrolytes, glucose, BUN, creatinine, liver transaminases, prothrombin time and ECG.
- Measurement of organic halogen compounds in urine is suggested to be an indicator of exposure.

Management

Pre-hospital

- Remove contaminated clothing and discard leather items.
- Wash affected skin, including hair and nails with copious amounts of water and soap.
- Irrigate eyes with copious amounts of tepid water or saline in case of eye exposure.
- In case of seizures put a spoon in the patient's mouth to prevent injury to tongue.
- Lay patient on side to prevent aspiration of vomitus.
- Do not induce vomiting.

- Do not give oil, milk or cream orally.
- Rescuers should avoid contact with contaminated clothing and vomitus.

Hospital

- Maintain the airway and assist ventilation if required. Administer supplemental oxygen.
- Perform gastric lavage and administer activated charcoal as a slurry in water or cathartic.
- Repeat dose activated charcoal may be beneficial.
- Give cathartics for gut decontamination.
- Do not give oil based cathartics.
- Control seizures with anticonvulsants.
- Treat recurrent seizures with phenobarbital.
- Give dopamine for resistant hypotension.
- Avoid epinephrine or atropine as they may lead to cardiac arrhythmias.
- Administer cholestyramine, a non-absorbable bile acid binding; anion exchange resin to all symptomatic patients.
- There is no specific antidote.

Carbamates

Carbamates are used widely as miticides, aphicides and insecticides in agriculture and veterinary practice. Many household sprays contain their formulation in petroleum distillates and are applied as spray droplet emulsions. Granular formulations are also available for agricultural use.

Common formulations
Aldicarb: Temik.

Carbaryl: Agroryl, Agrovin, Bangvin 50 WP, Dhanuvin 50 WP, Hexavin, Kevin 50, Kildiryl, Kilex carbaryl, Parryvin 50 WP, Sevidol, Sevin 50, Sujacarb, Sulfarl 50.

Carbofuran: Agrofuran, Curaterr, Diafuran, Furacarb, Furadan Carbocil, Furatox, Fury, Hexafuran, Yaltox.

Carbosulfan: Marshal.

Ethiofencarb: Arylmate, Croneton.

Fenobucarb: Baycarb, Bipvin.

Methiocarb: Draza, Mesurol.

Methomyl: Astra Lannate, Dunet, Dunil.

Propoxur: Baygon bait, Baygon flea collars, Baygon power aerosol, Baygon spray, Blattanex spray, Hit, Suncide.

Thiodicarb: Larvin.

Mechanism of toxicity

The mechanism of action is similar to OPs leading to excessive accumulation of acetylcholine at muscarinic, nicotinic and central nervous system receptors but they cause a short-lived reversible inhibition of acetylcholinesterase enzyme.

Most of them are poorly absorbed dermally as compared to OPs with the exception of aldicarb. They are absorbed by inhalation, ingestion and across the skin.

Toxic dose

The potency of carbamates is highly variable (Table 2).

Table 2. Classification of carbamates

Mild toxicity	Moderate toxicity	High toxicity
Carbaryl	Bufencarb	Aldicarb
Ethiofencarb	Carbosulfan	Aminocarb
Fenocarb (BPMC)	Dioxacarb	Carbofuran
Isoprocarb	Primicarb	Dimetilan
Metacrate	Propoxur	Isolan
	Thiodicarb	Methiocarb
	Trimethacarb	Methomyl
		Oxamyl

Clinical features

- Characteristic signs of exposure are salivation, lacrimation, urination, defecation, gastrointestinal distress and emesis (SLUDGE syndrome).
- Other signs and symptoms include miosis, headache, altered sensorium, dyspnea, rales, respiratory depression, chest tightness, bronchospasm, diaphoresis, bradycardia, hypotension, muscle twitching, tremors, paresthesias, cramping, weakness, tachycardia and pupillary dilatation.
- In severe poisoning respiratory depression, mental confusion, unconsciousness and convulsions may occur. Children are more susceptible to seizures than adults.
- Aspiration pneumonitis may be precipitated after ingestion of formulations in hydrocarbon vehicles.
- Inhalation of dusting powders causes laryngeal irritation, violent cough, diaphoresis and tachypnea.
- Death is rare and may be due to respiratory failure.

Diagnosis

Diagnosis is based on history of exposure and characteristic muscarinic, nicotinic and CNS signs and symptoms.

Laboratory/Monitoring

- Red blood cell cholinesterase and plasma cholinesterase are not reliable indicators of carbamate poisoning because of the rapid and spontaneous recovery of enzyme activity within several minutes or hours. However, depression of 25% or more from an individual's baseline value indicates exposure.
- Immediate analysis of sample is essential as *in vitro* hydrolysis of carbamates can occur.

Management

Pre-hospital

- Prehospital treatment remains the same as in the case of organophosphates.

Hospital

- Maintain the airway and assist ventilation if required.
- Perform gastric lavage and administer activated charcoal as a slurry in water or cathartic.
- Administer IV fluids.
- Give cathartics for gut decontamination.
- Control seizures with anticonvulsants.
- Treat recurrent seizures with phenobarbital.
- Avoid theophylline, succinylcholine and phenothiazines.
- Atropine is the specific antidote.
- Role of pralidoxime is controversial. However, it is indicated if there is (a) severe muscle weakness, fasciculations, paralysis or decreased respiratory effort (b) continued excessive requirement of atropine or (c) concomitant organophosphate and carbamate exposure.

Aluminium phosphide

Aluminium phosphide is a grain fumigant, used widely as a preservative by the northern wheat producing states of India. It is available as 3 g pellets which mainly contain 57% aluminium phosphide, rest being urea and ammonium carbamate. Each 3 g pellet releases 1 g of phosphine upon exposure to air. Phosphine is a colourless, flammable gas with an odour of garlic or rotten fish. Phosphine is used for fumigation, production of metal phosphides and in semiconductor industry.

Common preparations
Alphos, Celphos, Phosfume, Phosphotek, Phostox, Quickphos, Synfume.

Mechanism of toxicity

The exact mechanism of toxicity due to aluminium phosphide is not known. It causes cellular hypoxia due to non-competitive inhibition of mitochondrial cytochrome oxidase producing widespread organ damage. Further, disturbance in permeability of sodium, potassium, magnesium and calcium ions causing changes in transmembrane action potential in myocardium has also been proposed.

Toxic dose

The usual lethal dose in an adult is reported to be less than 500 mg. Inhalation of phosphine at a concentration of 200 ppm is considered immediately dangerous to life or health (IDLH).

Clinical features

- Mild poisoning due to ingestion causes epigastric distress, vomiting and diarrhea.
- In mild to moderate poisoning epigastric pain, vomiting, diarrhea, restlessness, hypotension (sys. BP < 90 mm Hg), tachycardia or bradycardia are observed. Cardiac arrhythmias and shock are the main findings. ECG abnormalities may include sinus tachycardia, sinus arrhythmias, ventricular premature complexes and ventricular tachycardia.
- Cough, dyspnea, adult respiratory distress syndrome, pulmonary edema and jaundice are also reported.
- CNS symptoms include fatigue, headache, restlessness, anxiety, drowsiness, dizziness, paresthesias and CNS depression.
- There is no change in the level of consciousness until late, though seizures may occur after acute exposure.
- Severe metabolic acidosis is common later in the course of poisoning.
- Hypomagnesemia, hypermagnesemia and hypokalemia may occur occasionally.
- Inhalation exposure causes severe pulmonary irritation, cough, dyspnea, headache, dizziness, lethargy and stupor. Gastroenteritis, seizures, renal and hepatic toxicity may also occur. The onset of symptoms is rapid, although delayed onset of pulmonary edema and focal myocardial necrosis has also been described.
- Observe all patients of inhalation for 72 hrs. for the signs and symptoms of delayed onset of pulmonary edema.
- Death is due to shock and peripheral circulatory failure.

Diagnosis

It is based on history of exposure, characteristic signs and symptoms and breath odour of decaying fish. Confirmation of diagnosis is done by qualitative test for the presence of phosphine in the gastric aspirate and breath.

Laboratory/Monitoring

- Monitor BUN, creatinine, potassium, magnesium, liver transaminases, arterial blood gases and chest X-ray.
- Monitor cardiac status continuously.

Management

Pre-hospital

- Move the patient immediately to fresh air and lay on side to prevent aspiration of vomitus.
- Give CPR if required and do not give mouth to mouth breathing.
- Induce emesis with syrup of ipecac.
- Shift the patient immediately to hospital.

Hospital

- Treatment is supportive and symptomatic.
- Provide adequate oxygenation and ventilatory support as required.
- Manage circulatory shock with IV fluids and give vasopressors if needed.
- Role of gastric lavage is controversial. However, an early gastric lavage with very dilute (1:10,000) potassium permanganate solution can be given.
- Activated charcoal as a slurry may be useful in adsorbing phosphine.
- Treat metabolic acidosis with sodium bicarbonate.
- Treat local irritation of GIT with H_2-receptor antagonists like ranitidine.
- Control seizures with anticonvulsants.
- Treat recurrent seizures with phenobarbital.
- Do not give diuretics at all in face of severe shock. However, a low dose of furosemide can be tried if the systolic blood pressure is > 90 mm Hg.
- Role of magnesium sulphate is controversial as there are no controlled studies to prove its efficacy. It has been successfully used in many studies with reduction in mortality.
- There is no specific antidote.

Pyrethrins and Pyrethroids

Pyrethrins are active insecticidal ingredients present in oleoresin extract of dried *Chrysanthemum* flowers. They are esters of pyrethric and chrysanthemic acids formed by the keto-alcohols pyrethrolone, cinerolone and jasmololone.

Pyrethrin I and pyrethrin II are the two most potent pyrethric and chrysanthemic ester insecticides. The synthetically derived compounds used as "insect knockdowns" are called pyrethroids which are subtly modifed to resist photolysis and to improve stability in the natural environment. Piperonyl butoxide is added to these compounds to increase their effectiveness and prolong the activity. Many pyrethrin-pyrethroid insecticides are formulated in petroleum distillates for spray applications and some are marketed in cans pressurized by propellants.

Common formulations

Allethrin: Baygon mats, Mortein power coil, Pynamin Forte, Sweet dream.

D-Allethrin: Baygon knockout aerosol, Baygon power mats, Good knight mosquito mats, HIT insect repellant.

Cypermethrin: Angel, Ankush, Agrocyper, Auzar, Baadha, Bilcyp, Basathrin, Blaze, Challanger, Cilcord, Colt 25, Cryux, Cybil, Cymbush, Cypercin, Cypermil, Cyperoid, Cyper, Cyperguard, Cyperhit, Cyperin, Cypermethrin, Cyper top, Cyrex, Cypersul, Sandoz, Cymet, Cypermar, Gilcyp Tech, Hilcyperin, Hi-power, Hycyper, Indothrin, Jawa, Lacer, Mortal, Panther, Parathrin, Piothrin, Polytrin, Ralathin, Ralothrin, Ripcord, Ramceper, Shakti, Sicerin, Simpler, Spec Cyperin, Starcyprin, Starcip, Super killer, Suraksha, Tackle, Trofy 25 EC, Ustad, Vegfrucolt, Volcyper, White gold.

Decamethrin: Decasyn, Decathrin.

Deltamethrin: Decis, Hexit, Lakshman rekha.

Fenvalerate: Fennock 20, Tictat.

Permethrin: Ambush, Hilthrin, Permasect.

Mechanism of toxicity
Both pyrethrins and pyrethroids have low mammalian toxicity. They paralyze the nervous system through disruption of membrane ion transport system in axons and pyrethroids prolong sodium influx and may also block inhibitory pathways. Low mammalian toxicity is primarily due to their rapid metabolic breakdown, ester cleavage and then rapid oxidation. Paresthesias caused by pyrethroids are due to the direct effect on intracutaneous nerve endings at very low doses. As very young children can not hydrolyze pyrethrum esters efficiently, they are more susceptible to poisoning. Both pyrethrins and pyrethroids are absorbed across the gut, pulmonary membrane and slightly across the intact skin.

Toxic dose
The toxic oral dose in mammals is greater than 100-1000 mg/kg and 10-100 g is potentially lethal. Ingestion of "Chinese chalk" used as an insect repellant containing 37.6 mg of deltamethrin per chalk is generally considered nontoxic.

Clinical features

- Ingestion causes salivation, nausea, vomiting, abdominal cramps, tenesmus, and gastritis.
- Neurological symptoms include paresthesias, headache, dizziness, choreoathetosis, fatigue and weakness. Massive exposure may result in hyperexcitability, seizures and coma.
- Large doses of concentrated formulations may cause coma (within 20 min.), fasciculations and seizures.
- Dermal exposure causes burning, tingling, itching and numbness.
- Irritant contact dermatitis is not common. Common lesion is erythematous dermatitis with vesicles, papules in most areas and intense pruritis. A bulbous dermatitis may develop.
- Inhalation commonly causes congestion, running nose and irritation in the throat.
- Hypersensitivity reactions and asthma like symptoms characterized by pneumonitis, cough, dyspnea, wheezing, chest pain and bronchospasm are observed.
- Rare cases of respiratory paralysis and cardiopulmonary arrest are reported.

Diagnosis

It is based on history of exposure. There are no specific laboratory tests or characteristic clinical symptoms which may help in their identification.

Laboratory/Monitoring

- Monitor electrolytes, glucose and arterial blood gases.
- Detection of parent compound is usually not useful because it is rapidly metabolized in the body.

Management

Pre-hospital

- Move the patient to fresh air from the source of exposure in case of inhalation and observe for any signs and symptoms of systemic toxicity.
- Wash affected skin with copious amounts of soap and water.
- Irrigate eyes with lots of tepid water.
- Do not induce vomiting.
- Consider prehospital administration of activated charcoal as an aqueous slurry in patients who are awake and able to protect their airway.

Hospital

- Treatment is supportive and symptomatic.
- Protect the airway. Give 100% humidified supplemental oxygen with assisted ventilation as required in case of inhalation.

- Administer activated charcoal and cathartics.
- Perform gastric lavage only after a potentially life threatening ingestion.
- Control seizures with anticonvulsants.
- Treat mild cases of anaphylaxis with antihistamines with or without epinephrine.
- Treat severe anaphylaxis with oxygen supplementation, aggressive airway management, epinephrine and IV fluids. Monitor ECG.
- Apply Vitamin E oil topically to relieve paresthesias.
- There is no specific antidote.

Ethylene dibromide

Ethylene dibromide (EDB) is a clear, heavy liquid with an odour of chloroform. It is used as an agricultural fumigant and industrial chemical. It is also used as a scavenger for lead in gasoline, in grain and crop fumigants and general solvents. EDB also finds use in waterproofing preparations, synthesis of dyes, pharmaceuticals and other brominated compounds, fire extinguishers and gauge fluids.

Mechanism of toxicity

Upon ingestion EDB is converted into active metabolites which get irreversibly bound to macromolecules including DNA, resulting in inhibition of enzymes. Oxidative (cytochrome P-450) and conjugation pathways (glutathione) are involved in the metabolism of EDB. The principal target organ of toxicity is liver.

Toxic dose

Ethylene dibromide is toxic following ingestion, inhalation and upon dermal contact. Ingestion of 4.5 ml of EDB has resulted in death. Death is also reported in a patient with a history of ethanol abuse with just 1.0 ml of EDB. Lung irritation is reported after exposure to vapour concentrations greater than 200 ppm and a concentration of 400 ppm may be immediately dangerous to life or health. However, no safe workplace exposure limit has been determined as EDB is a suspected carcinogen.

Clinical features

- Ingestion causes vomiting, diarrhea, headache, dizziness, weakness, fever, hypoglycemia, metabolic acidosis, shock, jaundice, oliguria, anuria, ventricular fibrillation, seizures and coma.
- In fatal cases, skeletal muscle necrosis, acute renal failure and hepatic necrosis are reported.
- Inhalation of vapours causes irritation of eyes, cough, pharyngitis, dyspnea, pneumonitis, pulmonary edema, cyanosis and respiratory depression.

- Pulmonary edema which usually occurs within 1-6 hrs. may be delayed upto 48 hrs. after exposure.
- Dermal exposure produces irritation, painful local inflammation, burning, redness and blistering.
- Death is usually due to hepatic failure, renal failure or respiratory depression.

Diagnosis

Diagnosis is based on history of exposure and evidence of gastroenteritis after ingestion and upper airway and eye irritation after inhalation.

Laboratory/Monitoring

- Monitor arterial blood gases, pulse oximetry, CBC, electrolytes, liver and renal function tests, blood glucose, urinalysis, serum calcium, phosphorous and magnesium levels.
- Monitor ECG, cardiac enzymes, chest X-ray and or coagulation profile in case of signs and symptoms of adverse cardiac, hematologic or pulmonary effects.

Management

Pre-hospital

- Move patient to fresh air in case of exposure by inhalation.
- Remove contaminated clothing and wash skin with copious amounts of water and soap.
- Do not induce emesis.
- Consider prehospital administration of activated charcoal in patients who are awake.

Hospital

- Treatment is supportive and symptomatic.
- Maintain the airway and assist ventilation if necessary. Give supplemental oxygen.
- Dilute with milk or water (120-240 ml) not exceeding 15 ml/kg in children.
- Perform gastric lavage in patients who present within 30 min. of ingestion or have ingested a large quantity and follow by activated charcoal and non oil based cathartic.
- Control seizures with anticonvulsants.
- Give antibiotics in case of infection.
- Role of corticosteroids in prevention of noncardiogenic pulmonary edema is not proven.
- There is no specific antidote.

Rodenticides

Zinc phosphide

It is a common rodenticide available as dark gray tetragonal crystals or as heavy, gray, crystalline powder which releases phosphine gas upon contact with dilute acids or water. The signs and symptoms of poisoning due to zinc phosphide are similar to aluminium phosphide characterized by gastrointestinal irritation, respiratory, circulatory, cardiac and cerebral impairment followed by renal and hepatic toxicity. The treatment is supportive and symptomatic. There is no specific antidote.

Barium carbonate

The water soluble salts of barium (acetate, carbonate, chloride, hydroxide, nitrate, sulphide) are highly toxic agents. The soluble salts are found in fireworks, depilatories and rodenticides. They are also used in the manufacture of glass and in dyeing textiles. Barium carbonate and chloride are used as pesticides and rodenticides. Barium carbonate is a white powder frequently mistaken for flour.

Mechanism of toxicity

Barium compounds produce neuromuscular blockade by persistent depolarization at neuromuscular junction. These salts also produce hypokalemia probably because barium ions have a direct action on muscle cell potassium permeability, which stimulates smooth, striated and cardiac muscles resulting in peristalsis, arterial hypertension, muscle twitching and cardiac arrhythmias.

Toxic dose

There is insufficient data to characterize accurately the acute toxicity of barium. The toxic dose of various barium salts may be as low as 200 mg and the lethal dose for most salts is 1-15 g.

Clinical features

- Initial features include nausea, vomiting, abdominal pain and diarrhea followed by headache, paresthesias and profound muscle weakness.
- Cardiovascular toxicity manifests itself as tachycardia and arrhythmias.
- Profound hypokalemia and skeletal muscle weakness develops progressing to flaccid paralysis of limbs and respiratory muscles.
- Acute renal failure and pulmonary dysfunction may also occur.
- Death may result from hypokalemia, arrhythmias, cardiac and respiratory failure.

Diagnosis

It is based on history of exposure accompanied by rapidly progressive hypokalemia and muscle weakness.

Laboratory/Monitoring

- Monitor electrolytes, BUN, creatinine and arterial blood gases.
- Monitor cardiac status for several hours after ingestion.

Management

Pre-hospital

- Induce emesis with syrup of ipecac.

Hospital

- Treatment is supportive and symptomatic.
- Maintain the airway and assist ventilation if required.
- Administer IV fluids.
- Perform gastric lavage with magnesium sulphate or sodium sulphate.
- Magnesium sulphate or sodium sulphate may be given orally to precipitate ingested barium salt as insoluble sulphate salt. Do not give IV magnesium sulphate.
- Treat hypokalemia with potassium chloride.
- Barium elimination may be enhanced by diuresis with saline and furosemide to obtain a flow of 4-6ml/kg/hr.
- There is no specific antidote.

Warfarin

Warfarin is widely used as a therapeutic anticoagulant and a rodenticide. This type of rodenticide contains only 0.025–0.050% warfarin and thus toxicity depends on repeated exposure.

Mechanism of toxicity

Warfarin acts by inhibiting vitamin-K dependent clotting factors (II, VII, IX, X) with consequent prolongation of prothrombin time and direct capillary damage. It is rapidly absorbed following ingestion and produces toxic effects by either large acute or smaller chronic ingestions. Warfarin is poisonous by ingestion, inhalation and intravenous route. It is moderately toxic by skin contact, subcutaneous and intraperitoneal routes.

Toxic dose

The lowest oral lethal dose reported in humans ranges from 6-15 mg/kg. Generally, a single, small ingestion of 10-20 mg does not cause serious intoxication. However, chronic or repeated ingestion of small amounts (2 mg/day) can produce significant anticoagulation.

Clinical features

- Common feature of poisoning is the asymptomatic prolongation of prothrombin time.

- Patients can present with bruising, hematuria, hemoptysis, malena, hematemsis and menorrhagia.
- Life-threatening complications include massive GI bleeding and intracranial hemorrhage.

Diagnosis

It depends on history of exposure and characteristic signs and symptoms. Confirmation can be done by measuring plasma prothrombin time.

Laboratory/Monitoring

- Quantify the anticoagulant effect by daily repeated measurement of prothrombin time which may not show elevation for 1-2 days. A normal prothrombin time (48-72 hrs.) post exposure rules out significant ingestion. A decrease in blood levels of clotting factors II, VII, IX, X can be noted. However, it is not routinely available.
- Other laboratory studies include CBC, blood group typing and cross match.

Management

Pre-hospital

- Do not induce emesis for single acute exposures.

Hospital

- Give activated charcoal and a cathartic.
- Avoid gastric lavage in patients already anticoagulated.
- Administer cholestyramine orally to enhance elimination.
- Treat small elevations in prothrombin time with vitamin K_1.
- Treat life-threatening hemorrhage with large doses of parenteral vitamin K_1 and infusion of fresh frozen plasma.
- Vitamin K_3 (menadione) K_4 are not effective.

Superwarfarins

Superwarfarins are potent long acting anticoagulants and include 4-hydroxy-coumarins (bromodiolone, brodifacoum, difenacoum) and indanediones (diphacinone, chlorophacinone, pindone). They produce a more potent and persistent anticoagulant effect than warfarin or other coumarin compounds.

Mechanism of toxicity

Superwarfarins cause a more effective blockade of vitamin K_1 epoxide cycle than warfarin. They also inhibit the synthesis of factors II, VII, IX, X in liver like warfarin but have a longer duration of action. They continue to produce significant anticoagulation for weeks to months after a single ingestion.

Toxic dose
These compounds have prolonged effects even after a single ingestion of 1 mg in an adult.

Clinical features

- Massive exposure produces hypoprothrombinemia and associated blood diathesis.
- Hemorrhage is the most common sign with epistaxis, gum bleeding, hemoptysis, hematuria, GI bleeding, bloody stools, abdominal and flank pain.
- Prolongation of prothrombin time starts between 36-48 hrs.
- Evidence of continuing anticoagulant effect may persist for days, weeks or even months.
- Cardiac and neurological features are produced with chronic ingestions of pindone.

Diagnosis
It is based on history of exposure and evidence of anticoagulant effect.

Laboratory/Monitoring

- Same as in case of warfarin. Daily repeated measurement of prothrombin time may not show elevation until 1-2 days after ingestion.
- Normal prothrombin time 48-72 hrs. post exposure rules out significant ingestion.

Management

Pre-hospital

- Induce emesis within 30 minutes of ingestion.

Hospital

- Admit patient for atleast 48-72 hrs. to detect clinical bleeding.
- Give vitamin K_1 (phytomenadione) in case of bleeding, after checking the prothrombin time.
- Give blood transfusion or fresh-frozen plasma in case of active hemorrhage.
- Do not precipitate hemorrhage by falls and other trauma in severely anticoagulated patients.
- Avoid drugs that enhance bleeding or decrease metabolism of the anticoagulant.
- Vitamin K_3 (menadione) is not effective.

Sodium fluoroacetate

Sodium fluoroacetate is a white, tasteless, odourless powder soluble in water. It is extremely toxic when ingested or inhaled and is a very effective rodenticide.

Mechanism of toxicity

Fluoroacetate is metabolized to the toxic compound fluorocitrate which blocks cellular metabolism by inhibiting the Kreb's cycle.

Toxic dose

Severe toxicity may be caused by as little as 1 mg of pure compound. Death is likely after ingestion of more than 5 mg/kg.

Clinical features

- Signs and symptoms may develop within 30 min. of exposure but may be delayed as long as 20 hrs.
- Manifestations include nausea, vomiting and diarrhea.
- Serious poisoning results in seizures, coma, respiratory depression, hypotension, cardiac arrhythmias including ventricular tachycardia, fibrillation and asystole.
- Metabolic acidosis, renal insufficiency, elevated transaminases, hypocalcemia and hyperacidosis are associated with an increased risk of fatal outcome.

Diagnosis

It is based on history of ingestion and clinical findings which may be delayed for several hours. Poisoning may mimic other cellular toxins like hydrogen sulphide or cyanide although the onset of symptoms is usually more rapid with these poisons.

Laboratory/Monitoring

- Monitor electrolytes, glucose, BUN, creatinine, arterial blood gases and chest X-ray.

Management

Pre-hospital

- Do not induce emesis.

Hospital

- Treatment is supportive and symptomatic.
- Precede gastric lavage by activated charcoal.
- Give an additional dose of activated charcoal and cathartic after performing gastric lavage.

- Administer IV fluids to enhance excretion, avoiding fluid overload.
- Control seizures with anticonvulsants.
- Give 10% calcium gluconate, IV slowly to relieve hypocalcemia.
- Monitor cardiac status continuously.
- There is no specific antidote.
- Safety and efficacy of glyceryl monoacetate and ethanol administration advocated to prevent or reverse the toxic effects of fluoroacetate has not been demonstrated in humans. Recent evidences have suggested that these experimental therapies are totally ineffective as fluoroacetate is rapidly incorporated in the Kreb's cycle, so it does not appear that these compounds have any antidotal effect.

Thallium
Thallium is an extremely toxic metal found commonly in fine dusts. The salts of toxicological importance are thallium sulphate and thallium acetate. Thallium sulphate is a highly toxic rodenticide. It is also used in industry and in homeopathic remedies. Thallium salts are used widely in the manufacture of optical lenses, photoelectric cells and costume jewellery.

Mechanism of toxicity
Thallium affects the mitochondria and a variety of enzyme systems resulting in generalized cellular poisoning. Because thallium metabolism has some similarities to that of potassium, it may inhibit potassium.

Toxic dose
The minimum lethal dose of thallium is 12 mg/kg body weight. It is a cumulative poison. The toxicity varies widely depending on the compound. Death is reported after ingestion of 3.29 mg of thallium sulphate. The more water soluble forms (sulphate, acetate, malonate, carbonate) are more toxic than the less water soluble forms (sulphide, iodide).

Clinical features
- Signs and symptoms usually appear within 12-24 hrs. post exposure.
- Ingestion results in metallic taste, dryness of mouth, soreness of gums, rhinorrhea, salivation, nausea, vomiting, bloody diarrhea, hematemesis, abdominal pain progressing to intestinal obstruction.
- Shock may result from massive fluid or blood loss.
- Neurological symptoms which appear within 2-5 days after exposure include headache, lethargy, muscle weakness, paresthesias, tremors, delirium, seizures and coma.

Diagnosis
It is based on history of exposure and presence of severe gastroenteritis.

Laboratory/Monitoring

- Monitor calcium levels, CBC, electrolytes, glucose, BUN, creatinine, hepatic transaminases, renal and cardiac functions closely.
- A 24 hr. urine quantitative assay is a reliable test.
- Concentrations greater than 100 μg/L are considered toxic (normal urinary thallium concentration is less than 1.5 μg/L).

Management

Pre-hospital

- Induce emesis within minutes of ingestion.
- Administer charcoal in patients who are awake and able to protect airway.

Hospital

- Treatment is supportive and symptomatic.
- Perform gastric lavage with 1% sodium or potassium iodide followed by activated charcoal and a cathartic.
- Repeat dose activated charcoal may enhance fecal elimination.
- Control seizures with anticonvulsants.
- Treat shock with IV fluids and vasopressors if required. Monitor fluid balance to avoid fluid overload.
- Give an infusion of potassium chloride to displace thallium from cells and accelerate excretion. However, the infusion may worsen encephalopathy so the patient should be monitored carefully.
- Combine hemodialysis and hemoperfusion to achieve moderate reduction of body burden in severely poisoned cases.
- Give prussian blue (potassium ferric ferrocyanide) via a naso jejunal tube and continue therapy till the urinary excretion of thallium is less than 0–10 μg/24 hrs.
- British antilewisite (BAL) and other chelators have also been tried with varying success.
- There is no specific antidote.

Strychnine

Strychnine is a white, crystalline, very bitter alkaloid obtained from the seeds of *Strychnos nux vomica*. It is used in tonics, cathartics, analgesics, sedatives and stimulants and veterinary products. However, its use in pharmaceutical preparations is restricted and at present it is used as a rodenticide and a common adulterant of street drugs like cocaine and marijuana.

Mechanism of toxicity

Strychnine competitively antagonizes glycine, an inhibitory neurotransmitter released by post synaptic inhibitory neurons in the spinal cord causing increased neuronal excitability resulting in generalized seizure like contraction of skeletal muscles. It is absorbed rapidly from the gut and nasal mucosa.

Toxic dose

An oral fatal dose of 16 mg is reported, though deaths have been reported with much less amounts also. Infact, it is difficult to establish a toxic dose and any dose should be considered life threatening.

Clinical features

- Signs and symptoms occur within 15-30 min. of ingestion and include bitter taste, restlessness, muscular stiffness, painful cramps followed by generalized muscle contractions and opisthotonos. Muscle contractions are easily triggered by physical or emotional stimuli and are intermittent.
- True seizures are not caused but muscle contractions and may resemble the tonic phase of a grand mal seizure. The patient is awake and painfully aware of contractions.
- Hyperalgesia, increased visual stimulation and hyperacusis' may be caused. Muscle contractions may also be triggered by sudden noises and other sensory inputs.
- Rhabdomyolysis, hyperthermia, metabolic acidosis, myoglobinuria and renal failure often result due to repeated and prolonged muscle contractions.
- Death is due to respiratory arrest or secondary to hyperthermia or rhabdomyolysis and renal failure.

Diagnosis

It is based on history of ingestion and presence of generalized muscle contractions (seizure like) accompanied often by metabolic acidosis, hyperthermia and rhabdomyolysis.'

Laboratory/Monitoring

- Monitor electrolytes, BUN, creatinine, CPK and arterial blood gases.
- Monitor urine for occult blood which is positive in presence of urine myoglobinuria.
- Toxic serum strychnine concentration is 1 mg/L, although blood levels do not correlate well with the severity of toxicity.

Management

Pre-hospital

- Do not induce emesis.

- Limit external stimuli (noise, touch, light).
- Shift the patient to hospital.

Hospital

- Maintain the airway and assist ventilation if required.
- Perform gastric lavage in large ingestions.
- Administer activated charcoal and cathartic.
- Control muscle spasms with anticonvulsants or barbiturates.
- Treat hyperthermia and rhabdomyolysis.
- Give sodium bicarbonate for metabolic acidosis.
- In severe cases administer pancuronium to produce complete neuromuscular paralysis.
- There is no specific antidote.

Yellow phosphorous

Yellow phosphorous is a wax-like crystalline solid with garlic like odour and is almost insoluble in water. It ignites spontaneously upon contact with air at or above 30°C and explodes to oxidizing materials, releasing primarily phosphorous sesquioxide. It is soluble in fats and bile and is absorbed from the intestine and subcutaneous injections especially when administered in a finely divided form. It is used in the manufacture of rodenticides, incendiaries, phosphorous compounds and pyrotechnics and as a semiconductor additive. In the past, it was used in the manufacture of matches causing both acute and chronic poisoning after ingestion of matches.

Mechanism of toxicity

Phosphorous is a general protoplasmic poison. It may cause extensive fatty degeneration of liver, kidneys, brain and other organs of the body.

Toxic dose

The estimated acute lethal adult dose by ingestion is 1 mg/kg. Severe symptoms have been reported in an adult after ingestion of 15 mg. As little as 3 mg has been reported to cause death in a two year old child.

Clinical features

- Initial GI effects after ingestion are followed by a relatively asymptomatic period lasting for 8 hrs. to several weeks terminating in acute liver and renal failure with metabolic derangements.
- Ingestion causes burning pain in throat, chest and abdomen followed by nausea, vomiting, diarrhea and hematemesis. The vomitus is smoking luminescent with a garlicky odour.
- CNS symptoms include restlessness, irritability, drowsiness, lethargy, weakness, delirium, stupor and coma.

- GI symptoms may be accompanied by cardiovascular collapse.
- Metabolic derangements may occur including hypocalcemia and hyperphosphatemia (or hypophosphatemia).
- Death in first 12 hrs. is usually the result of peripheral vascular collapse and within 24-48 hrs. may ensue from peripheral vascular collapse frequently accompanied by acute renal failure.

Diagnosis

It is based on history of exposure and clinical presentation. "Smoking" and luminescent stools and vomitus suggest phosphorous ingestion.

Laboratory/Monitoring

- Monitor CBC, platelet count, electrolytes, liver and renal function tests, urinalysis, urine output, ECG, serum calcium and phosphorous, International normalized ratio or prothrombin time.
- The onset of hepatic and renal involvement is often delayed for at least 24 hrs. and mandates a period of observation.

Management

Pre-hospital

- Do not induce emesis because of its corrosive potential.
- Administer activated charcoal in awake patients.
- Wash the exposed skin burns with copious amounts of water.

Hospital

- Treatment is supportive and symptomatic.
- Role of gastric lavage is controversial in view of its potential corrosive effects and potential for perforation. However, gastric lavage with potassium permanganate (1:5,000 soln.) may be done as it converts phosphorous into harmless oxidation products.
- There is no specific antidote.

Alpha-chloralose

Alpha chloralose is a rodenticide used in the control of bird pests and to kill mice, rats and moles. It is available as baits containing 1.5 and 4% alpha chloralose. Ingestion is unlikely to cause toxicity unless a large quantity has been consumed. The oral toxic dose is reported to be 1-4 g and 20 mg/kg in adults and children respectively. Acute toxic ingestions result in sedation, coma, respiratory depression, myoclonic or generalized seizures and hypotension. Paradoxically, it possesses both depressant effects producing sedation and anaesthesia as well as a stimulant action. Gastrointestinal symptoms like abdominal pain and vomiting are also seen. Treatment is supportive and symptomatic and there is no specific antidote.

Alpha-naphthyl thiourea

It is a blue-gray, odourless, slightly bitter powder which is used as a rodenticide, as baits in concentrations of 1-3%. Ingestion is not expected to result in significant human toxicity. However, large doses may produce pulmonary edema and hypothermia. Management of poisoning involves supportive and symptomatic treatment.

Cholecalciferol

It is a rodenticide available as pellets containing 0.075% cholecalciferol (2300 units of vit. D). Its ingestion may be acutely toxic. Emesis, activated charcoal and cathartics are seldom necessary in acute ingestion unless extremely large amounts are ingested. Calcium levels need to be monitored continuously. Chronic ingestion causes toxicity resulting in hypercalcemia which leads to anorexia, nausea, vomiting, diarrhea, drowsiness, fatigue and weight loss. Polyuria, polydypsia, proteinuria and azotemia result from acute renal tubular injury. Coma may occur in severe cases. Treatment is supportive and symptomatic. Perform gastric lavage. Repeated administration of activated charcoal may be useful.

3. Herbicides and Fungicides

Herbicides

Herbicides are compounds that have the potential of either killing or damaging unwanted plants or weeds. Herbicides may be categorized into various groups on the basis of their chemical nature (Table 1).

Table 1. Common herbicides

Common herbicides	Examples
Dinitrocompounds	Dinitro orthocresol (DNOC), dinitrophenol (DNP) pentachlorophenol (PCP) etc.
Phenoxyacetic acids	2,4-dichlorophenoxyacetic acid, 2,4,5-trichlorophenoxyacetic acid
Bipyridium compounds	Diquat, paraquat etc.
Heterocyclic compounds	Atrazine, propazine, simazine etc.
Chloroaliphatic acids	Dalapon, sodium chloroacetate, sodiumtrichloroacetate etc.
Substituted ureas	Monouron, diuron, isoproturon, metoxuron, diflubenzuron, metribuzin etc.
Substituted dinitroanilines	Pendimethalin etc.

Dinitrocompounds

Dinitrophenols

Dinitrophenols are substituted phenols used as insecticides and herbicides. They are relatively insoluble in water. Commercial products are dissolved in organic solvents and used for spray applications. Some wettable powder formulations are also available.

Dinitrophenol has been used as a spray against aphids and mites, as a fungicide and a wood preservative against various moulds and mildews and sometimes as a weed killer. It is used as an intermediate for manufacturing dyes and photographical agents. 2,4-dinitrophenol was used for stimulation of metabolism and promotion of weight loss long back, however, its use for this purpose has been banned now-a-days.

Mechanism of toxicity

Toxicity due to these compounds is attributed to their ability to uncouple oxidative phosphorylation. This results in the inefficient use of energy and development of hypermetabolic state.

Toxic dose

The oral fatal dose in adults is 1-3 g. A dose of 3 g has proven fatal even in divided doses over a period of 5 days.

Clinical features

- Early symptoms include thirst, headache, confusion, malaise and lassitude.
- Systemic poisoning causes hyperthermia, tachypnea, extreme diaphoresis, metabolic acidosis, abnormally yellow coloured urine and stool.
- Liver and kidney damage may ensue within 12 to 72 hrs. post exposure.
- Seizures, coma, cyanosis, pulmonary edema and arrhythmias may be observed.
- Methemoglobinemia may also occur in some cases.

Diagnosis

It is based on history of exposure, clinical findings and characteristic signs and symptoms of poisoning.

Laboratory/Monitoring

- Monitor fluids and electrolytes.
- Monitor glucose, arterial blood gases, liver and renal function tests in symptomatic patients.

Management

Pre-hospital

- Do not induce emesis.
- Administer activated charcoal as an aqueous slurry in patients who are awake and have protected airway. It is most effective when administered within 1 hr. of ingestion.
- Reduce body temperature with sponge baths.

Hospital

- Provide supportive care and decontaminate.
- Ensure a clear airway by nasopharyngeal suction of secretions/vomitus.
- Administer oxygen by mechanically assisted pulmonary ventilation to minimize tissue anoxia.
- Administer activated charcoal and a cathartic.
- Treat seizures with anticonvulsants.

- Atropine is absolutely contraindicated as it is essential not to confuse the manifestations of dinitrophenol poisoning with that of cholinesterase inhibition.
- There is no specific antidote.

Pentachlorophenol

Pentachlorophenol (PCP), a substituted phenol is a synthetic, lipophilic substance that is commonly used as a fungicide, herbicide, defoliant and wood preservative. It is also used to prevent fungal rot and decay.

Mechanism of toxicity

Pentachlorophenol acts as a cellular poison by uncoupling oxidative phosphorylation. The consequent increase in metabolic rate leads to excessive heat production or hyperthermia. The main route of exposure is inhalation and ingestion.

Clinical features

- Acute exposure causes irritation of skin, eyes and respiratory system.
- Systemic absorption may cause headache, vomiting, weakness and lethargy.
- In fatal poisoning profound sweating, hyperthermia, tachycardia, tachypnea, convulsions and coma may occur.
- Pulmonary edema is also reported.
- Death is usually due to cardiovascular collapse or hyperthermia.

Diagnosis

It is based on history of exposure and clinical findings and should be suspected in a patient with fever, metabolic acidosis, diaphoresis and tachypnea.

Laboratory/Monitoring

- Monitor CBC, electrolytes, BUN, creatinine and CPK.
- Monitor urine dipstick for occult blood, arterial blood gases and liver transaminases, methemoglobin levels and chest X-ray.
- Estimate urinary levels. Levels less than 36ppm are usually not associated with significant symptoms.
- Monitor blood levels. Levels greater than 1 mg/L indicate excessive exposure.

Management

Pre-hospital

- Do not induce emesis because of the potential for CNS depression and seizures.

Hospital

- Perform gastric lavage.
- Administer activated charcoal and a cathartic.
- Manage hyperthermia by sponging with tepid to cool water.
- Do not give atropine, aspirin or other salicylates to control hyperthermia as they tend to enhance the toxicity of PCP.
- Manage hypotension with intravenous fluids and use vasopressors if required.
- Treat seizures with anticonvulsants.
- There is no specific antidote.

Phenoxyacetic acids

Phenoxyacetic acids are used as herbicides. They are used to control broad-leaf weeds and woody plants. The water soluble esters are formulated as aqueous solutions and less water soluble esters are used as emulsions. There are many commercial formulations available which include 2,4-D (2,4-dichlorophenoxyacetic acid), 2,4,5-T (2,4,5-trichlorophenoxyacetic acid), MCPA (methyl chlorophenoxy acetic acid), MCPP (4-chloro-2-methyl phenoxypropionic acid).

Mechanism of toxicity
Chlorophenoxy compounds are weak uncouplers of oxidative phosphorylation.

Toxic dose
The minimum toxic dose of 2,4-D in humans is 3-4 g or 40-50 mg/kg on body weight basis. Fatalities due to 2,4-D have been reported after ingestion of amounts ranging from 80 mg/kg to 3 g/kg. An amount of 814 mg/kg of MCPA is the lowest reported oral fatal dose.

Clinical features

- Acute ingestion may cause miosis, vomiting, abdominal pain, diarrhea, headache, confusion, fever, hypotension, tachycardia, bradycardia and ECG abnormalities.
- Muscle rigidity, pulmonary edema, possible respiratory failure and rhabdomyolysis may occur.

Diagnosis
The diagnosis depends on history of exposure, presence of muscle weakness and elevated CPK.

Laboratory/Monitoring

- Obtain baseline CBC, platelet counts and electrolytes.

- Monitor hepatic and renal function tests, alkaline phosphatase, CPK, arterial pH and sodium bicarbonate.
- Monitor urine for pH, proteins, RBC's myoglobin and urinary output.

Management

Pre-hospital

- Induce emesis with syrup of ipecac.

Hospital

- Treatment is supportive and symptomatic
- Perform gastric lavage.
- Administer activated charcoal and cathartics.
- Manage hypotension with intravenous fluid.
- Treat seizures with anticonvulsants.
- Administer sodium bicarbonate to render urine alkaline.
- Monitor the patient closely for atleast 6-12 hrs. after ingestion because of the potential for delayed onset of symptoms.
- There is no specific antidote.

Bipyridium compounds

Paraquat

Paraquat is a quaternary bipyridyl, nonspecific contact herbicide available as colourless crystals (dichloride salt) or a yellow solid (bis-methyl sulphate salt). It has a faint ammonia-like odour and is soluble in water. Technical products are available as liquids with concentrations ranging from 20-50%. Paraquat has been previously used to destroy illicit marijuana plants.

Mechanism of toxicity

Paraquat causes lipid peroxidation and subsequently cell death.

Toxic dose

The estimated lethal dose is 3-5 mg/kg or 10-15 ml of a 20% w/v solution of paraquat. Ingestion of 20-40 mg of paraquat ion per kg body weight (7.5-15.0 ml of 20% w/v concentrate) results in death in most cases, which may be delayed upto 2-3 weeks, while ingestion of more than 40 mg of paraquat ion per kg body weight (>15.0 ml of 20% w/v concentrate) results in mortality in essentially all cases within 7 days.

Clinical features

- Ingestion of <20 mg/kg of paraquat may cause oral mucosal ulceration, nausea, vomiting and diarrhea.

- Ingestion of higher doses may cause sore throat, difficulty in swallowing, abdominal pain and GI distress.
- At higher doses progressive pulmonary fibrosis developing over 3-14 days may lead to respiratory failure and death 2-4 weeks post ingestion.
- Renal damage indicated by proteinuria and hematuria commonly appears within first 24-96 hrs. It may progress to acute tubular necrosis. Acute glomerulonephritis has been reported.
- Ingestion of 60 ml of concentrated solution may cause death within 24 hrs.
- Massive gastroenteritis, corrosive esophageal injury, pulmonary edema and cardiogenic shock may occur.

Diagnosis

It is based on history of ingestion and presence of characteristic features. The oral mucosa burns may have the appearance of a pseudomembrane on the soft palate which resembles that of diphtheria.

Laboratory/Monitoring

- Monitor electrolytes, glucose, renal and liver functions, baseline urinalysis and urine output.
- Monitor pulmonary function tests and chest X-ray.
- Obtain arterial blood gases serially for several days.

Management

Pre-hosptial

- Remove patient from source of exposure to fresh air.
- Remove contaminated clothing.
- Wash affected skin with copious amounts of water and soap.
- Irrigate eyes with lots of tepid water.
- Avoid direct contact with contaminated clothing and vomitus. Members of the rescue team should wear rubber gloves while washing pesticide from skin and hairs.

Hospital

- Provide supportive and symptomatic care.
- Maintain the airway and assist ventilation if necessary.
- Avoid excessive oxygen administration in patients with paraquat poisoning, as it may aggravate lipid peroxidation reactions in the lungs.
- Treat significant hypoxemia with supplemental oxygen, using only the lowest oxygen concentration necessary to achieve a PO_2 of about 60 mm.

- Administer IV fluids to combat hypotension. Vasopressors should be given in refractory hypotension.
- Perform gastric lavage.
- Administer Fuller's Earth or Bentonite. Administer repeated doses of activated charcoal at 4 hrs. intervals.
- Give cathartic. Repeat dose of cathartic if adsorbent does not appear in stool within 6 hrs. of administration.
- Treat seizures with anticonvulsants.
- There is no specific antidote.

Diquat

Diquat dibromide is available commercially as an aqueous solution (15-25% w/v) and as water soluble granules. It is a highly ionized molecule poorly absorbed through intact human skin.

Mechanism of toxicity

The concentrated solution of diquat is corrosive. It does not cause pulmonary fibrosis but instead causes gastrointestinal fluid sequestration, renal failure, cerebral and brain stem hemorrhagic infarction.

Toxic dose

The estimated minimum lethal dose in an adult (60 kg) is 25 ml of the concentrate (240 mg ion/ml × 25 ml = 6,000 mg diquat ion or 100 mg/kg). Ingestion of more than 90 ml affects all organ systems resulting in death within 24 to 48 hrs.

Clinical features

- Ingestion or absorption, of concentrated diquat solution, through damaged skin may result in systemic toxicity.
- Ingestion of approximately 90 ml of concentrate or less, causes an initial burning sensation of the oral and pharyngeal mucosa.
- Nausea, repeated vomiting and abdominal discomfort (pain following diarrhea) are noted depending upon the amount ingested.
- Gastrointestinal distress may persist for 2 to 3 days. Transient irritation and ulceration of the oral mucosa may be evident by this time.
- Larger doses can also produce ulcerations of the digestive tract, pulmonary edema, acute liver and kidney failure, and rapid loss of consciousness.
- Death occurs from multiorgan failure.
- Concentrated solutions can cause severe eye irritation.

Diagnosis

It is based on history of exposure alongwith characteristic signs and symptoms. The diagnosis can be confirmed by performing qualitative and quantitative tests.

Laboratory/Monitoring

- Determine baseline renal function tests, if exposure is significant enough to cause systemic poisoning.
- Monitor BUN and creatinine, 10 to 12 hrs. post ingestion.

Management

Pre-hospital

- Do not induce emesis.
- Administer activated charcoal preferably within 1 hr. as an aqueous slurry in patients who are awake and able to protect their airway.

Hospital

- Provide supportive and symptomatic treatment.
- Support respiratory and cardiovascular functions.
- Control seizures with anticonvulsants.
- Monitor for respiratory depression, hypotension, arrhythmias, and the need for endotracheal intubation.
- Evaluate for hypoxia, electrolyte disturbances and hypoglycemia.
- Treat pain associated with mucosal ulceration with analgesics.
- Carefully observe patients with inhalation exposure for the development of any systemic signs and symptoms and provide symptomatic treatment as necessary.
- There is no specific antidote.

Heterocyclic compounds

Atrazine

Atrazine, the most widely used triazene herbicide is a selective herbicide for crops like maize, sorghum, sugarcane, pineapple etc. Triazine herbicides are structurally and toxicologically similar to triazoles. Amitrole is a synonym for triazole. Triazines are incorporated into many herbicidal mixtures for special applications. The technical concentrates are sprayed as emulsions in organic solvents.

Mechanism of toxicity

The mechanism by which these agents produce toxicity is not well understood.

Toxic dose

Most triazines exhibit low systemic toxicity in laboratory rodents and farm animals. Very low mammalian toxicity is reported. Ingestion of 800 mg of atrazine in a child and 4 mg/kg in an adult has not resulted in toxicity.

Clinical features

- Adverse effects of triazine in humans have not been reported.
- Symptoms such as anorexia, salivation, depression of activity, muscle spasms and fasciculations, ataxia, increased body temperature and dyspnea are reported after ingestion of atrazine in cattle.
- Ocular and skin irritation may occur following triazole exposure.

Diagnosis

It is based on history of exposure and clinical signs and symptoms.

Management

Pre-hospital

- Do not induce emesis.

Hospital

- Provide supportive and symptomatic treatment.
- There is no specific antidote.

Chloroaliphatic acids

The most commonly used chloroaliphatic acids are dalapon, sodium chloroacetate and sodium trichloroacetate. These agents are relatively harmless. Dalapon is a selective translocated herbicide used for grass weed control. The most common source of poisoning is accidental ingestion. Sheep and goats are the frequently affected animals.

Mechanism of toxicity

Dalapon is a chlorinated hydrocarbon insecticide and is an "axon poison".

Clinical features

- Anorexia, lassitude, diarrhea and mild cyanosis are commonly observed symptoms.

Management

- Provide supportive and symptomatic treatment.
- There is no specific antidote.

Substituted ureas

Substituted urea herbicides are photosynthesis inhibitors used mainly for weed control in non-crop areas. This class of herbicides includes chlorimuron, neburon, monuron, diuron, metobromuron, tebuthioron, tetrafluron and isoproturon which are the commonly used substituted ureas having low toxicity potential. Poisoning with these agents is rare.

Mechanism of toxicity
Diuron is well absorbed from the GI and respiratory system, but information about dermal exposure is not available. It undergoes hepatic metabolism and majority of the metabolites are excreted in urine. Monuron has also been shown to undergo metabolism via liver microsomes.

Toxic dose
There is insufficient data to accurately assess the minimal toxic or lethal dose. On the basis of animal studies, these agents appear to have a low order of systemic toxicity.

Clinical features
- Severity of intoxication is assessed on the basis of clinical findings.
- Methemoglobinemia may be noted in large ingestions.

Laboratory/Monitoring
- Obtain a baseline CBC, renal and hepatic function tests, including urinalysis for protein and cells.
- Plasma levels are not clinically useful.
- Obtain methemoglobin levels in all cyanotic patients and patients demonstrating dyspnea or other signs of respiratory difficulty.

Management

Pre-hospital
- Induce emesis within an hour with syrup of ipecac.

Hospital
- Support respiratory and cardiovascular functions.
- Methylene blue is the specific antidote for methemoglobinemia.

Substituted dinitroaniline compounds

Pendimethalin and trifluralin are the substituted dinitroaniline compounds having a broad spectrum weedicide activity and low mammalian toxicity. Trifluralin is available as 25% and 44% emulsifiable concentrate and 2.5-10% granules.

Toxic dose
Minimum lethal human exposure is unknown.

Clinical features
- Trifluralin is irritating to eyes and produces mild skin irritation after prolonged exposure.

- Adverse effects in humans have not been described.
- Massive overdose results in CNS depression.

Management

Pre-hospital

- Do not induce emesis because of the potential for CNS and respiratory depression.
- Administer activated charcoal as an aqueous slurry in patients who are awake and able to protect their airway. It is most effective when administered within one hour of ingestion.

Hospital

- Provide supportive and symptomatic treatment.
- Observe intoxicated patients carefully for the possible development of esophageal or GI irritation or burns.
- Consider endoscopy if signs and symptoms of esophageal irritation or burns are suspected.
- Irrigate exposed eyes with copious amounts of tepid water for at least 15 min. If irritation persists, consult an ophthalmologist.
- There is no specific antidote.

Fungicides

Fungicides are effective against fungi. Mercury (Hg) compounds mainly used as fungicides are mercurial salts and organic mercurial compounds. Common fungicides are categorised into phthalimide, benzimidazole and carbamate groups (Table 2).

Table 2.   Common fungicides

Common fungicides	Examples
Phthalimides	Captan, Captafol
Benzimidazole	Benomyl
Dithio Carbamates	Thiram, Ziram, Zineb, Nabam, ETU, Maneb, Mancozeb

Phthalimide fungicides

The phthalimide fungicides are frequently mixed with other commonly used insecticides, such as diazinon and lindane. Captan, captafol and folpet are widely used fungicides and seed protectants. Captan is used as a preservative in cosmetics. Captafol is a white, crystalline solid with pungent odour and used as a fungicide on fruits and vegetables.

Mechanism of toxicity

The phthalimide fungicides are metabolized in the liver. Captan is an alkylating agent.

Toxic dose

Acute toxicity by usual routes of exposure to phthalimide fungicides is not known.

Clinical features

- Major phthalimide fungicides (captan, folpet, and captafol) have similar spectrum of toxicity.
- Folpet is a respiratory tract irritant and can produce occupational asthma.
- Nausea and vomiting with diarrhea may occur following ingestion of Captan in large quantities.
- Other than irritant action, allergic dermatitis, conjunctivitis and respiratory sensitization, no other signs of toxicity in humans are reported.

Diagnosis

The diagnosis is based on history of exposure.

Laboratory/Monitoring

- No specific laboratory tests are generally necessary unless indicated by the clinical presentation.

Management

Pre-hospital

- Induce emesis within 30 min. of ingestion.
- Administer activated charcoal.

Hospital

- Provide supportive and symptomatic care.
- Administer 100% humidified supplemental oxygen with assisted ventilation as required.
- Perform gastric lavage.
- Control seizures with anticonvulsants.
- No specific treatment is necessary in most cases, but observe the patient for toxicity and treat symptomatically as indicated.
- Observe the patient with inhalation exposure carefully for the development of any systemic signs and give symptomatic treatment as necessary.
- Flush exposed skin/eyes with copious amounts of water.

Benzimidazoles

Benomyl

Benomyl is a white crystalline solid, insoluble in oils, usually available in the form of a wettable powder, for application to a wide range of vegetables, fruits and field crops. In aqueous solutions, it decomposes to carbendazim and an ethyl analog. Benomyl has also been used in veterinary medicine as an anthelmintic, against mites and an oxidizer in sewage treatment.

Mechanism of toxicity

There is little evidence of benomyl toxicity in mammals, probably largely due to its limited absorption. It is a benzimidazole carbamate fungicide with a low degree of toxicity. Exposure is not associated with signs and symptoms of cholinergic stimulation.

Toxic dose

The minimum toxic or lethal dose in humans is unknown.

Clinical features

- Systemic symptoms have rarely been reported following exposure.
- It may be irritating to eyes, skin and mucous membranes. Contact dermatitis has been reported after exposure.
- Benomyl may cause sensitization in some people.

Laboratory/Monitoring

- Benomyl plasma levels are not clinically useful or readily available.
- No specific laboratory work is needed unless otherwise clinically indicated.

Management

Pre-hospital

- Administer activated charcoal as an aqueous slurry in patients who are awake and able to protect their airway.
- After inhalation exposure move patient from source of exposure.

Hospital

- Treatment is supportive and symptomatic.
- Support respiration if required.
- There is no specific antidote.

Carbamate fungicides

The dithiocarbamates are an important group of fungicidical agents. They are chemically related to the carbamate insecticides. In addition, thiram, ziram and ferbam are related to disulfiram. The solutions, suspensions or emulsions of carbamate fungicides are applied as sprays. Thiram is the methyl analogue of disulfiram and is an important agricultural fungicide. Thiram is used for foliage and seed treatment, as a disinfectant for nuts, fruits, and mushrooms. Ethylene thiourea (ETU) is used as an accelerator, in rubber vulcanization, dyes and synthetic resins.

Mechanism of toxicity
Thiram and carbamate compounds are metabolized in part, to carbon disulphide. This may be one of the mechanisms whereby these chemicals are neurotoxic at extraordinary dosage.

Toxic dose
Systemic toxicity of these compounds is generally low.

Clinical features
- Unlike the carbamate insecticides, the dithiocarbamate fungicides do not have anticholinesterase activity. Exposure to these agents does not result in cholinergic symptoms.
- Systemic poisoning by these agents has been very rare.
- If ingested, these agents are likely to cause nausea, vomiting and diarrhea.
- Respiratory effects may be seen secondary to aspiration of the solvent.
- Confusion, drowsiness, lethargy may occur after poisoning with thiram.
- Toxicity is compounded in association with hydrocarbon based solvents.

Laboratory/Monitoring
- Blood levels are not clinically useful.
- Monitor arterial blood gases, electrolytes and blood glucose.

Management

Pre-hospital
- Do not induce emesis.

Hospital
- Provide supportive and symptomatic care.
- Provide ventilatory support if needed.
- Perform gastric lavage. In case of sustained release formulations and

substances known to form bezoars or concretions, lavage can be given more than 60 min. after ingestion.

- Administer charcoal as an aqueous slurry.
- Evaluate for hypoxia, electrolyte disturbances and hypoglycemia.
- Give intravenous fluids in case of profuse vomiting and diarrhea.
- Monitor for respiratory depression, hypotension, arrhythmias and the need for endotracheal intubation.
- Control seizures with anticonvulsants.
- There is no specific antidote.

Mercury compounds

Organic mercury (Hg) compounds are mainly used as antiseptics/antibacterials, fungicides, herbicides, mild weedicides, seed disinfectants and as preservatives in pharmaceuticals. Most of the organic mercury compounds are crystals, granules, scales or powders, which may be incorporated into other preparations. Organic mercury compounds are further divided into three classes: (a) aryl compounds are phenyl mercuric salts which are used to prevent fungal growth on seeds (b) methoxy methyl mercuric chloride and methoxy ethyl mercuric acetate are used as fungicides (c) alkyl compounds. Organic mercury compounds have been used in veterinary practice.

Mechanism of toxicity

Organic mercurials comprise of aryl, long and short chain alkyl compounds. Replacement of hydrogen ion in sulfhydryl group by mercury causes widespread dysfunction of enzymes, transport mechanisms, membrane and structural proteins. The metal also reacts with carboxylic, amide and phosphoryl groups. Volatile organic mercury compounds like methyl mercury are readily absorbed across the pulmonary mucosal membrane and may lead to respiratory distress.

Toxic dose

The estimated average lethal dose of organic mercury compounds in general, is 100 mg.

Clinical features

- Ingestion leads to GI symptoms.
- Methoxy ethyl mercury compounds are primarily associated with gastrointestinal, renal and neurological toxicity.
- Predominant CNS signs and symptoms include tremors, headache, numbness, fatigue and difficulty in thinking.
- Incoordination, slurred speech, loss of position, sense and hearing, constriction of visual fields are observed in severe poisoning.
- Renal tubular dysfunction and ECG abnormalities have been observed.
- Dermatitis has also been reported.

Diagnosis

The diagnosis is based on their blood levels.

Laboratory/Monitoring

- Obtain 24 hr. urine for estimation of mercury.
- Monitor baseline BUN, creatinine, electrolytes and perform urinalysis.
- Obtain whole blood mercury levels for recent acute exposures.

Management

Pre-hospital

- Wash skin and hair contaminated by mercurial dust or solutions thoroughly with soap and water.
- Move patient of inhalation exposure immediately to fresh air.
- Induce emesis with syrup of ipecac.

Hospital

- Provide supportive care.
- Provide endotracheal intubation and ventilatory support if required.
- Perform gastric lavage with milk followed by normal saline.
- Give IV fluids.
- Administer activated charcoal.
- In methyl mercury intoxication, limited data suggests that oral DMSA may be effective in decreasing Hg levels in tissues, including the brain.
- Do not give BAL in poisoning by metallic or organic mercury as it may redistribute mercury to the brain from other tissue sites.
- D-penicillamine has been shown to increase urinary mercury excretion and decreases blood mercury levels in patients poisoned with methyl mercury.

Copper compounds

Copper compounds are used in insecticides, fungicides and algicides. Copper is a lustrous, ductile, malleable, odourless solid with distinct reddish or reddish brown colour. In water the colour of copper is often blue or green. When exposed to moist air, copper gradually develops a coating of green basic carbonate. Copper sulphate is used as a fungicide, wood preservative, for water treatment, as a bactericide, algaecide and a molluscicide. Common copper compounds are listed in Table 3.

Mechanism of toxicity

Copper compounds are well absorbed after ingestion, inhalation and through skin. Systemic absorption can produce hepatic and renal tubular injury.

Table 3.   Common copper compounds

Generic name	Trade name
Copper acetoarsenite	Paris green
Cuprous oxide	Cuprous oxide
Copper oxychloride	Bongcop, Copper force, Cuprastar, Cuprosol, Agro coxy, Blue copper, Blue diamond, Blitox copen, Ramcop sucop, Quintozene
Copper sulphate	Copper sulphate

Toxic dose

Ingestion of more than 250 mg of copper sulphate produces vomiting. Large ingestions cause hepatic and renal injury. Ingestion of 10 g of copper sulphate has resulted in death.

Clinical features

- Ingestion causes metallic taste, epigastric burning, vomiting and diarrhea, with the subsequent development of gastric ulceration and hemorrhage.
- Hemolysis, hemoglobinuria and jaundice may also occur.
- Copper dust causes respiratory irritation leading to sore throat and cough.
- Inhalation of copper oxide leads to systemic toxicity, manifested as "metal fume fever".
- Dermal absorption of copper compounds causes contact dermatitis. Greenish-blue discoloration of skin is caused by excessive dermal exposure.
- Early deaths are due to shock while hepatic and renal failure are responsible for delayed death.

Diagnosis

Diagnosis is based on the history of exposure and characteristic signs and symptoms.

Laboratory/Monitoring

- Obtain whole blood copper levels.
- Monitor baseline liver and renal function tests and CBC.

Management

Pre-hospital

- Remove contaminated clothing.
- Wash affected skin with soap and lots of water.
- Induce emesis with syrup of ipecac.

Hospital

- Ensure a clear airway by nasopharyngeal suction of vomitus/secretions.
- Administer IV fluids to prevent shock.
- Give gastric lavage with lukewarm water or saline.
- Chelation therapy with D-penicillamine may be useful especially when renal insufficiency is not present.
- BAL is the specific antidote for copper poisoning.

4. Heavy Metals

Arsenic

Arsenic is found both in pentavalent and trivalent forms in organic and inorganic compounds. Trivalent salts (arsenite) are more toxic than the pentavalent (arsenate) ones. Both organic and inorganic arsenic compounds are used extensively as herbicides, fungicides, weedicides (lead arsenate), rodenticides, insecticides (sodium arsenite, copper arsenite) and wood preservatives. In industry, they are used in glass manufacturing, pigment production, hardening of copper, lead, alloys and in semiconductors. Arsenic compounds are used in veterinary pharmaceuticals, Indian and Chinese folk remedies, homeopathic medicines and misused as a contaminant of "moonshine" whisky.

Mechanism of toxicity

There is disruption of enzymatic reactions which are vital to cellular metabolism by arsenic compounds. The arsenites interact with the sulfhydryl group while arsenates substitute for phosphate. Soluble arsenic compounds are well absorbed after ingestion or inhalation. Inorganic arsenic dusts like arsenic trioxide cause systemic poisoning after percutaneons absorption.

Toxic dose

The arsenic compounds vary in their toxicity based on the physical state, solubility, animal species involved and valence state. Generally trivalent arsenic (As^{3+}) is 2–10 times more toxic than the pentavalent form (As^{5+}). The fatal dose of trivalent form like sodium arsenite could be as little as 100-300 mg.

Clinical features

- Gastrointestinal symptoms occurring within minutes of acute exposure include nausea, vomiting, abdominal pain, watery diarrhea (rice water stools), burning sensation and dryness of mouth and dysphagia. A garlic odour of breath may be present.
- Fluid loss and extensive tissue third-spacing of fluids from gastroenteritis may lead to hypotension, shock and death.

- Cardiac manifestations include cardiomyopathy, hypotension, prolonged QT interval and non-specific ST-T changes, ventricular fibrillation or tachycardia, and non-cardiogenic or cardiogenic pulmonary edema.
- Hypovolemic or hemorrhagic shock may occur.
- CNS symptoms include delirium, altered sensorium, encephalopathy and coma. Delayed sensorimotor peripheral neuropathy occurs 2–6 weeks after acute ingestion.
- In moderate poisoning, usually early painful dysesthesia occurs while in severe poisoning ascending weakness and paralysis may predominate. Peripheral neuropathy begins as paresthesias of the soles of feet, then the hands progressing proximally over the next few days. Severe muscle weakness and disability ensue. The symptoms may initially mimic Gullian-Barre syndrome.
- Severe poisoning is characterized by fever, delirium, seizures, hypotension, arrhythmias, pulmonary edema, respiratory failure, hemolytic anemia, acute renal failure and coma resulting in death.
- Acute hemolysis, decreased hematocrit may be observed.
- Hematuria, proteinuria, anuria, acute tubular necrosis, chronic renal insufficiency and renal failure are observed.
- Rhabdomyolysis may also occur.
- Dermal manifestations include flushing, diaphoresis, facial and peripheral edema, diffuse pruritic macular rash and brawny, non-pruritic desquamation. Aldrich-Mees lines which are transverse white striae in the nails are seen 2–4 weeks after acute poisoning.

Diagnosis

It is based on history of exposure and a typical presentation (abrupt onset of abdominal pain, vomiting, watery diarrhea, hypotension possibly in association with multisystem signs and symptoms). However, garlic-like odour of breath may not be always present. Blood levels of arsenic are highly variable. Arsenic concentration exceeding 50 µg/L or greater in 24 hr. urine specimen and concentrations of >1000 µg/L (spot urine, first 2–3 days) indicate exposure. Lower solubility compounds are opaque and may be visible in abdominal X-ray.

Laboratory/Monitoring

- Nail and hair levels exceeding more than normal level (<1 ppm) indicate exposure.
- Monitor CBC, electrolytes, glucose, BUN, creatinine, liver enzymes, CPK, urinalysis, and smear for basophilic stippling.
- Monitor ECG.
- Obtain abdominal and chest X-ray.

Management

Pre-hospital

- Induce emesis within minutes of ingestion.
- Move the patient to hospital.

Hospital

- Provide supportive treatment.
- Perform gastric lavage for large ingestions.
- Administer activated charcoal and cathartics.
- Administer IV fluids.
- Give vasopressors if volume replacement does not reverse hypotension.
- Treat arrhythmias avoiding use of class Ia antiarrhythmics (quinidine, disopyramide, procainamide etc.) and most class III drugs (N-acetyl procainamide, sotalol).
- Control seizures with anticonvulsants.
- Hemodialysis may be beneficial in patients with concomitant renal failure.
- Administer BAL, the specific antidote immediately in symptomatic patients.
- Dimethyl succinic acid (DMSA) has been found effective in pediatric poisoning.
- D-penicillamine can also be tried as a chelating agent.
- Observe patients closely for cardiopulmonary complications which may be delayed for several days.

Lead

Lead, a naturally occuring metallic element occurs in several mineral forms as galena (lead sulphide), anglisite (lead sulphate), cerussite (lead carbonate), mimetite (lead chloroarsenate), pyromorphite (lead chlorophosphate) etc. Common sources are industrial effluents, solders, lead paints, rubber toys, illicit whisky, ayurvedic and folk remedies and lead containing soldering fluxes. Lead is used as an ingredient in pigments for paints, enamels, ceramic glazes and glass, ingredients in plastics and rubber, metallurgy, foils, storage batteries, shielding for X-ray and atomic radiations and cable sheathing. Organic lead (tetra-ethyl and tetra-methyl) are added to gasoline as antiknock compounds. Exposure to tetraethyl lead is mostly due to purposeful inhalation of leaded gasoline.

Mechanism of toxicity

Lead affects the nervous system, the kidneys, reproductive and hematopoietic systems. It could cause alterations in cellular and mitochondrial membranes, neurotransmitter synthesis and function, heme synthesis and nucleotide metabolism. It inhibits enzymatic processes. It has a high affinity for metalloenzymes with sulfhydryl groups and also interacts with essential cations like zinc, calcium and iron. Tetraethyl lead is converted into triethyl and inorganic lead in the body which cause toxicity.

Toxic dose

Gastrointestinal absorption depends on chemical structure, solubility, particle size, GI transit time, nutritional status and chronologic age. There is 10% absorption in adults and 40% in children of ingested lead. Absorption of inhaled lead depends on vapour versus particle size and concentration. Intoxication has been reported after ingestion of several grams of lead acetate or tetraethyl lead remaining in intestinal tract for many days. The oral dose associated with lowest observable effect level (LOEL) in humans is uncertain, but oral ingestion of 20 μg/kg/day is reported to increase the levels from 15 μg/dl to 40 μg/dl in a 21-day chronic ingestion study along with an increase in erythrocyte protoporphyrin. Acute ingestion of 15 g of lead oxide has caused death. The level considered immediately dangerous to life or health after inhalation is 700 mg/m^3. The permissible exposure limit for tetraethyl lead is 0.07 mg/m^3 and its IDLH is 40 mg/m^3.

Organic alkyl compounds are absorbed rapidly and extensively after dermal absorption, but there is minimal dermal absorption of inorganic lead.

Clinical features

- Acute ingestion of acid-soluble lead compounds or inhalation of lead vapours causes toxicity.
- Ingestion of large amounts may cause thirst, metallic taste, nausea, anorexia, abdominal pain, vomiting, diarrhea or constipation, malaise, convulsions and shock.
- Paresthesias, pain and muscle weakness may occur.
- Kidney damage and oliguria are reported.
- Anemia, hemoglobinuria and toxic hepatitis may occur.
- Exposure to tetraethyl lead is commonly due to purposeful inhalation. Acute poisoning may occur due to ingestion, inhalation or dermal absorption. Symptoms occur within 1–5 days and as long as 14 days after exposure.
- CNS effects may occur together with the effects of solvent.
- Mild toxicity causes anxiety, irritability, insomnia, dizziness, metallic taste, ataxia, nausea, vomiting, pallor and mild diarrhea. Ingestion of large amounts may cause thirst, metallic taste, nausea, anorexia and abdominal pain.
- Moderate toxicity leads to disorientation, hyperexcitability, tremors, twitching, chorea, increased reflexes, bradycardia, hypotension, hypothermia, rotary or horizontal nystagmus.
- Delusions, hallucinations, mania, seizures, cerebral edema, coma and death occur in severe poisoning.

Diagnosis

Lead poisoning should be considered in any patient with multisystem findings of abdominal pain, headache and anemia. Renal insufficiency, gout and motor neuropathy are less common. Delirium or convulsions in children may suggest lead encephalopathy. Transiently high values of whole blood lead suggest acute exposure (normal blood levels are less than 10 µg/dl). Increase in free erythrocyte protoporphyrin (FEP) or zinc protoporphyrin (ZPP) from >35 µg/dl indicates lead induced inhibition of heme synthesis. A high blood lead level in presence of normal FEP or ZPP suggests recent exposure. Abdominal X-ray may show lead paint flakes or bullets. Other nonspecific diagnostic findings include anemia, basophilic stippling of erythrocytes and increased urinary coproporphyrin and aminolevulinic acid. In acute organic lead poisoning, urinary lead levels are raised with normal blood levels and erythrocyte porphyrin is slightly elevated. Anemia and basophilic stippling is rare.

Laboratory/Monitoring

- Monitor blood lead levels.
- Obtain CBC to assess anemia and perform a peripheral smear.
- Basophilic stippling and hypochromia suggest lead intoxication, but they are nonspecific and their absence does not rule out diagnosis.
- Monitor abdominal X-ray which reveals lead containing paint or objects as radio opacities.

Management

Pre-hospital

- Move patient to fresh air in case of inhalation exposure.
- Induce emesis with syrup of ipecac.
- Emesis is contraindicated following ingestion of leaded gasoline or products containing organic lead compounds.

Hospital

- Provide supportive and symptomatic care.
- Administer 100% humidified supplemental oxygen with assisted ventilation if required.
- Perform gastric lavage.
- Administer activated charcoal and cathartics.
- Consider whole bowel irrigation, repeated cathartics or enemas if X-ray shows lead containing material after initial treatment.
- Remove lead containing bullets, shrapnel or buckshot lodged in or adjacent to synovial spaces surgically, particularly in case of systemic lead absorption.
- Treat seizures with anticonvulsants.

- Mannitol or steroids may be tried for increased intracranial pressure.
- Administer IV fluids avoiding overhydration.
- Treat symptomatic intoxication without encephalopathy with DMSA or parenteral calcium EDTA.
- D-Penicillamine is an alternative treatment with more side effects and less efficacy.
- Give BAL and calcium EDTA if evidence of encephalopathy exists.

Mercury

Mercury, a naturally occurring metal exists in three forms i.e elemental (metallic) mercury, inorganic mercury salts (mercurous and mercuric salts) and organic mercury (alkyl mercury). Its various forms are chiefly used in the chloralkali production, paints and pigments, electrical equipment, dental amalgams, thermometers, gold mining and extracting batteries, topical antiseptics and disinfectants, fungicides, germicides, photography, tanning, embalming, wood preservatives or stains, herbicides, pesticides, catalysts, chemical intermediates, herbal medications etc. The inorganic mercury compounds were previously used as diuretics, antibacterials, antispetics, ointments and laxatives. However, many of these have been replaced by other therapeutic agents. Organic compounds mainly include aryl and alkyl mercury compounds. The aryl compounds are degraded into inorganic form in the body whereas the alkyl compounds (ethyl or methyl mercury) retain their forms. Mercurochrome and thiomersal are still used as topical antiseptics. Inorganic mercury is converted by organisms into methylmercury resulting in bioaccumulation.

Mechanism of toxicity
Mercury binds to the sulfhydryl groups causing widespread dysfunction of enzymes, transport mechanisms, membranes and structural proteins. Metallic mercury vapours are absorbed well after inhalation. Absorption from GIT and skin is limited. Inorganic mercury salts are generally corrosive.

Toxic dose
Chemical pneumonitis may occur at levels in excess of 1 mg/m^3 and airborne exposure to 28 mg/m^3 is considered immediately dangerous to life or health. Liquid metallic mercury has a very low gastrointestinal absorption and causes poisoning only in presence of abnormal gut motility or after peritoneal absorption. The acute oral lethal dose of mercuric chloride is approximately 1-4 g. Peritoneal lavage fluids containing 0.2-0.8% mercuric chloride have caused severe toxicity and death. Ingestion of 10-60 mg/kg of methyl mercury may be lethal. It has a significant oral absorption and is absorbed well after inhalation, ingestion and probably by dermal route.

Clinical features

Elemental mercury

- Metallic mercury vapours affect primarily the respiratory system. Main symptoms after inhalation include dyspnea, chest tightness, cough, necrotizing bronchiolitis, pneumonitis, pulmonary edema.
- GI symptoms include nausea, vomiting, metallic taste in the mouth, anorexia, abdominal pain and diarrhea.
- Rashes are common.
- Lethargy, weakness, chills, fever, headache and visual disturbances may occur.
- Renal damage and acute gingivostomatitis may also occur.
- Thrombocytopenia, anemia and lymphopenia are rare.

Inorganic mercury

- Inorganic salts are generally corrosive. Acute ingestion causes salivation, metallic taste in mouth, abdominal pain, nausea, vomiting, bloody diarrhea, dysphagia, hematemesis, proteinuria and nephrotic syndrome.
- Tachycardia, hypotension, potentially fatal hypovolemic shock and circulatory collapse, tremors, confusion, loss of coordination, hyper reflexia and lethargy may occur.
- Aspiration following ingestion may result in pulmonary irritation, pulmonary edema and adult respiratory distress syndrome.
- Dermal exposure can result in systemic toxicity.
- Acute tubular necrosis may develop within 48 hrs. after significant ingestion. Uremia, acute renal failure and death may result.

Organic mercury

- Short-chain alkyl mercury compounds (methyl mercury) primarily cause CNS effects which include tremors, headache, ataxia, fatigue, dysarthria, numbness and tingling of digits and face, paresthesias, tunnel vision and difficulty in thinking, hearing impairment, progressive chorea, athetosis and coma.
- Ethyl mercury may also cause gastroenteritis and renal damage.
- Phenyl mercury compounds cause symptoms intermediate between alkyl and inorganic mercury.

Diagnosis

It involves history of exposure, characteristic findings and presence of increased blood mercury levels or urinary excretion. Blood mercury levels of >20–50 µg/dl indicate acute exposure.

Laboratory/Monitoring

- Monitor 24 hrs. urine and blood for mercury levels.
- Monitor baseline BUN, creatinine, urinalysis, electrolytes, liver functions and arterial blood gases.
- Urine mercury levels are not useful in methyl mercury exposure. Whole blood mercury levels greater than 20 µg/dl are associated with symptoms.
- Monitor urinary markers of nephrotoxicity (microalbuminuria, β_2-microglobulin, retinol binding protein, N-acetylglucosaminidase).
- Monitor abdominal X-ray.

Management

Pre-hospital

- Move patient to fresh air in case of inhalation.
- Do not induce emesis in case of ingestion of inorganic salts or metallic mercury.
- Give milk or egg yolk for inorganic salt ingestion.
- Wash contaminated skin and hair with copious amounts of water.
- Irrigate eyes with lots of water.

Hospital

- Provide supportive care.
- Maintain the airway and assist ventilation if required.
- Metallic mercury passes through the intestinal tract with minimal absorption. Gut decontamination is not recommended.
- Consider whole bowel irrigation, repeat-dose cathartics therapy in case of large ingestion, intestinal perforation or abnormally diminished bowel motility.
- Surgical removal may be required if it is trapped in the intestine.
- Perform gastric lavage and administer activated charcoal for inorganic salts or organic mercury ingestion.
- Administer IV fluids.
- Dialysis may be required as a supportive treatment of renal failure.
- DMSA is the specific antidote for metallic mercury.
- DMPS (2,3-dimercaptopropane sulfonate) may be tried.
- Penicillamine is an alternative chelator.
- Administer BAL for inorganic mercury salts ingestion followed by DMSA.
- Limited data suggests effectiveness of oral DMSA in organic mercury poisoning (methyl mercury).
- BAL is not recommended in both organic and metallic mercury poisoning.

5. Household Products

Camphor

Camphor, a volatile organic compound with a distinctive pungent odour and taste, is used in many household products, usually at low concentrations. It is derived from the wood of the tree, *Cinnamomum camphora* or is synthesized from turpentine oil. It is a colourless or white compound in the form of crystals, granules or a translucent mass. Camphor has been used as an antipruritic and topical rubefacient, aphrodisiac, abortifacient, contraceptive, cold remedy, suppressor of lactation and antiseptic. It is an excellent plasticizer for cellulose esters and ethers. It is used in the manufacture of plastics, especially celluloid, in lacquers and varnishes, explosives, embalming fluids, as a moth repellent, and as a preservative in pharmaceuticals and cosmetics.

Mechanism of toxicity

Camphor is a central nervous system stimulant and causes seizures shortly after ingestion. The underlying mechanism is unknown. It is rapidly absorbed from the gastrointestinal tract and is metabolized by the liver. Camphor is rapidly oxidized to camphorol and then conjugated in liver to glucuronide form which is excreted in the urine. The metabolism may be responsible for the transient alterations in certain liver function tests.

Toxic dose

As little as 0.75 g of camphor, or one teaspoon of camphorated oil can be fatal to a child. One gram has caused death in a small child. In adults, 2 g can produce toxic symptoms, however, there are exceptions suggesting that even 20 g may be compatible with survival. Lethal dose is reported to be 50 to 500 mg/kg (5 ml of 100% camphor for a 10 kg toddler). Acute camphor poisoning secondary to tasting (or accidental ingestion of small amounts, i.e. one teaspoonful) of vicks vaporub, or similar products, is unlikely. An adult has survived a dose of as high as 30 g.

Clinical features

- It rapidly produces GI irritation and seizures following ingestion.
- Burning in mouth and throat occurs immediately, followed by nausea and vomiting.

- Ataxia, drowsiness, confusion, restlessness, delirium, muscle twitching and coma may occur.
- It typically causes abrupt onset of seizures about 20-30 min. after ingestion.
- Death may result from CNS depression and respiratory arrest.
- In rare cases, camphor poisoning may produce urinary retention, anuria, albuminuria, mild hepatic damage and mydriasis.
- Inhaling smoke of camphor may cause tracheobronchitis.

Diagnosis

Diagnosis is based on history of exposure and abrupt onset of seizures shortly after ingestion. The pungent odour of camphor and other volatile oils is usually apparent.

Laboratory/Monitoring

- Monitor electrolytes, glucose, arterial blood gases (if the patient is comatose or in status epilepticus) and liver function tests.

Management

Pre-hospital

- Do not induce emesis.
- Administer activated charcoal.

Hospital

- Provide supportive treatment.
- Support respiratory and cardiovascular functions.
- Maintain the airway and assist ventilation if required.
- Perform gastric lavage.
- Monitor for respiratory depression, hypotension and dysrhythmias.
- Evaluate for hypoxia, electrolyte disturbances and hypoglycemia.
- Administer IV fluids.
- There is no specific antidote.

Naphthalene

Naphthalene occurs naturally in the essential oils of the roots of *Radix* and *Herbaononidis*. It occurs naturally in crude oil from which it may be directly recovered as white flakes. It is derived from the distillation of coaltars and catalytic processing of petroleum.

Naphthalene may exist as a powder, cubes, spheres, or flakes. It is used commonly as a moth repellant in the form of balls, disks or flakes and as an ingredient in air freshener and toilet bowl deodorizers. It has been used in dusting powders for skin diseases and as an antiseptic and antihelminthic.

Naphthalene is used as a chemical intermediate and raw material for production of indigo and other dyes and in the production of naphthol and halogenated naphthalenes. It is also used in the manufacture of insecticides, fungicides, wood preservatives and synthetic resins.

Mechanism of toxicity

Naphthalene causes gastrointestinal upset and central nervous system stimulation. It may produce hemolysis, especially in patients with glucose-6-phosphate dehydrogenase (G-6-PD) deficiency.

Toxic dose

The minimum lethal dose of naphthalene is not known but ingestion of 2 g has produced death in G-6-PD deficient patients (one mothball is about 0.5 to 3.6 g). In non G-6-PD deficient patients, this amount is well tolerated.

Clinical features

- Other features include sweating, headache and confusion.
- Infants and patients with G-6-PD deficiency, sickle cell anemia, or sickle triat are more likely to develop hemolysis and methemoglobinemia.
- In severe cases, coma with or without convulsions may develop.
- Methemoglobinemia, hyperkalemia, fever, anemia and acute renal failure could occur.
- Intoxication can occur after dermal or inhalation exposure also. Hypersensitivity dermatitis is commonly observed after dermal exposure.
- Eye exposure to an airborne concentration of 15 ppm causes irritation. Eye contact with solid material may result in conjunctivitis, superficial injury to the cornea, diminished visual acuity, and other effects. It may cause cataracts.

Diagnosis

Diagnosis is usually based on history of ingestion and characteristic "mothball" odour around the mouth and in the vomitus.

Laboratory/Monitoring

- Obtain baseline CBC, electrolytes, G-6-PD level, liver and renal function tests, urinalysis and urine dipstick test for hemoglobinuria.
- Monitor methemoglobin levels in cyanotic patients.
- Abdominal X-ray may help differentiate between mothballs or other products which contain p-dichlorobenzene (densely radiopaque) from those which contain naphthalene (radiolucent or faintly radiopaque).

Management

Pre-hospital

- Induce emesis with syrup of ipecac immediately after exposure.
- Do not administer milk, fats or oils, which may enhance absorption.

Hospital

- Treatment is supportive and symptomatic.
- Maintain the airway and assist ventilation if required.
- Perform gastric lavage even in patients presenting late after ingestion.
- Administer activated charcoal and a cathartic.
- Treat coma and seizures if they occur.
- If laboratory findings are negative and the patient is asymptomatic for 4 to 6 hrs. post ingestion, the patient may be discharged with instructions for a follow-up, and CBC and urinalysis for upto 5 days post ingestion.
- Treat methemoglobinemia (> 30%) or those patients with signs other than cyanosis, with methylene blue.
- Blood transfusion, alkaline diuresis and corticosteroids may be beneficial in case of severe hemolysis.
- There is no specific antidote.

Kerosene

Kerosene is an aliphatic hydrocarbon and a simple petroleum distillate. Aliphatic mixtures such as gasoline, naphtha, mineral spirit, kerosene, thinner, furniture polish are poorly absorbed from the gastrointestinal tract. Kerosene has a low viscosity, low surface tension and high volatility. Kerosene oil is used to fuel stoves.

Mechanism of toxicity

Toxicity from hydrocarbons may be caused due to direct injury from pulmonary aspiration, or systemic intoxication after ingestion, inhalation or skin absorption.

Toxic dose

Risk of systemic toxicity after ingestion is low as long as it is not aspirated. Aspiration of just 0.2 ml may produce severe chemical pneumonitis. Recovery has been reported following ingestion of 250 ml.

Clinical features

- Kerosene oil ingestion generally produces an immediate burning sensation in the mouth and pharynx, as well as nausea and vomiting. In absence of aspiration, about 40–60 ml/kg of kerosene can be tolerated without any systemic effects.

- Aspiration can produce chemical pneumonitis. Depending upon severity, the picture varies from mild tachypnea and coughing to dyspnea, cyanosis and pulmonary edema, fever (with infection) and leukocytosis.
- CNS depression, hypoxia, drowsiness, convulsions and coma are reported.
- Fatalities occur primarily because of pulmonary complications. In rare cases, patients may develop ventricular arrhythmias.
- Inhalation may produce dyspnea, fever and severe hypoxia. These features resolve spontaneously.
- Intravenous doses of kerosene may produce acute apnea and cyanosis and later, pulmonary edema and pulmonary infiltrates.

Diagnosis

Diagnosis is based on history of exposure and presence of respiratory symptoms such as coughing, choking and wheezing. If these symptoms are not present within 4–6 hrs. of exposure, it is very unlikely that chemical pneumonitis will occur. Chest X-ray and arterial blood gases or oximetry may assist in the diagnosis of chemical pneumonitis. For systemic intoxication, diagnosis is based on a history of ingestion or inhalation, accompanied by systemic clinical manifestations.

Laboratory/Monitoring

- Monitor arterial blood gases.
- Monitor ECG, chest X-ray and pulmonary function tests in symptomatic patients.

Management

Pre-hospital

- Do not induce emesis because of the risk of aspiration.
- In case of inhalation, move the victim to fresh air.
- In case of dermal exposure, remove all contaminated clothing and wash skin with copious amounts of water.

Hospital

- Provide supportive care to symptomatic patients.
- Evaluate and maintain the ventilatory status.
- Administer supplemental oxygen.
- Do not perform gastric lavage due to the risk of aspiration.
- Avoid use of epinephrine and isoproterenol as they may precipitate ventricular arrhythmias.
- There is no specific antidote.

Phenol and related agents

Phenol (carbolic acid) is a disinfectant which exists as a weak acid. Chlorinated phenol derivatives are much less toxic than pure phenol. Phenol is available as technical products in fused (82%), crystal (90%) or liquid (95%) forms.

It can be obtained from the distillation of coaltar. It is used in explosives, fertilizers, paints, resins and disinfectants and primarily in the manufacture of bisphenol A, alkyl phenols, other chemicals and drugs. It is also used as a dye and indicator, medical and veterinary antiseptic, disinfectant, local anesthetic, preservative for parenteral medications, household cleaner, chemical face-peeling agent, and over-the-counter topical medication (skin and throat sprays). Other related products included are dinitrophenol, benzenol, hydroquinone and hydroxyquinone.

Mechanism of toxicity

Phenol denatures proteins and penetrates tissues well. It is a potent irritant that may cause corrosive injury to the eyes, GIT and respiratory tract. Systemic absorption causes central nervous system stimulation. The mechanism of CNS intoxication is not known. Some phenolic compounds (dinitrophenol and hydroquinone) may induce methemoglobinemia.

Toxic dose

The minimal toxic dose of phenol and related compounds is not well established. Acute ingestion of as little as 1 g of pure phenol in adults has resulted in death. Toxicity may be noted at significantly lower doses. Despite multiple complications, an adult recovered from an oral ingestion of 300 ml of 50% (150 g) cresol-soap solution.

Clinical features

- Phenol toxicity occurs most frequently following acute ingestion or chronic dermal application, however, systemic toxicity can also result from inhalation of vapours.
- Ingestion of concentrations greater than 5% may cause caustic GI burns and upper airway edema.
- Large ingestions or inhalation exposure may cause CNS depression, seizures, coma, hypotension and tachycardia.
- Systemic manifestations of toxicity include nausea, vomiting, diarrhea, dyspnea, profuse sweating, hypotension, arrhythmias, agitation, lethargy, methemoglobinemia and hemolytic anemia.
- Liver and renal injury may also occur.
- Dermal exposure causes lesions which are initially painless white patches and later turn erythematous and finally stain brown.
- Eye exposure may result in irritation, corneal injury and burns.

Diagnosis

Diagnosis is based on history of exposure, presence of a characteristic odour, and painless white skin burns.

Laboratory/Monitoring

- Obtain CBC, electrolytes and urinalysis.
- Obtain baseline liver and renal function tests. Consider daily monitoring for hepatocellular injury even after a 24 hr. asymptomatic period.
- Monitor acid-base balance closely.
- Obtain methemoglobin levels to detect methemoglobinemia after dinitrophenol or hydroquinone exposure.
- Perform endoscopy after ingestion of solutions of phenol with concentrations above 5% to assess severity of burns, or in patients with drooling, stridor, or persistent vomiting.

Management

Pre-hospital

- Irrigate exposed skin or eyes with copious amounts of water.
- Dilute with milk or water (120-240 ml) in case of ingestion.
- Do not induce emesis.

Hospital

- Consider gastric lavage for large ingestions.
- Administer one dose of activated charcoal without a cathartic in case substantial ingestion has occured within the previous few hours. However, it should be avoided if endoscopy is planned.
- Control convulsions with anticonvulsants.
- Monitor hemodynamics and pulmonary functions continuously.
- Administer methylene blue in case methemoglobin levels are greater than 30%.
- Manage metabolic acidosis with sodium bicarbonate.
- For inhalation exposure, administer 100% humidified oxygen and provide assisted ventilation if required.
- Dialysis does not increase the rate of excretion of phenol.
- There is no specific antidote.

Caustics and Corrosives

Acids

Any chemical causing tissue injury to the gastrointestinal tract and mucus membranes when ingested is treated as 'caustic'. Caustics may be divided into alkalies and acids. Acids produce coagulation necrosis of the gut mucosa and unless the agent is unusually strong or the contact prolonged, the formation of eschar limits the damage to superficial layers, while alkalies cause liquefactive necrosis of esophagus with saponification and continued penetration into underlying tissues causing extensive damage.

Acids are used in a variety of household products like toilet bowl cleaners, metal cleaners, antirust compounds, battery fluid and pool sanitizers. Industrial uses of concentrated acids include electroplating, photography, leather tanning, bleaching, printing and rayon manufacturing. Acidic caustic substances include phosphoric acid, sulphuric acid, oxalic acid, nitric acid and chromic acid. Acetic acid is used as a disinfectant and hairwave neutralizer. Concentrations of 5–10% are weak and irritant and more than 50%, corrosive. Vinegar is <5% acetic acid. Chromic acid is used in photography, electroplating and tanning. Oxalic acid is used for removing writing from the paper. It is a common household remedy for removing ink and rust stains from linen. Hydrochloric acid less than 5% is a weak irritant, 5% to 10% is strong irritant and more than 10% is corrosive. Sulphuric acid is used as a toilet, drain and metal cleaner. Concentrations of greater than 10% are corrosive. Phosphoric acid is used in metal cleaning and disinfectants. Concentrations of 15% to 35% are weak irritants, 35% to 60% are strong irritants and more than 60%, corrosive. Nitric acid 5% is used in engraving and in some gun barrel cleaners. Concentrations of more than 5% are corrosive.

Mechanism of toxicity
Acids are corrosive which may produce severe burns upon contact and gastrointestinal burns if ingested. The effect on tissues is a coagulation-type necrosis, causing destruction of surface epithelium and submucosa, with involvement of blood vessels and lymphatics.

Toxic dose
The toxic dose varies tremendously with the type and concentration of the acid. Phosphoric acid as little as 8 ml may be fatal if ingested. Ingestion of 15 ml of hydrochloric acid may be fatal. Acute ingestion of 5 g of oxalic acid has caused death. The mean lethal dose for an adult is probably about 15 to 30 g. Death may occur within a few hours.

Ingestion of 3–5 ml of glacial acetic acid may cause death but 200 ml of vinegar may not be harmful. A few drops of concentrated sulphuric acid and 5 ml of nitric acid may cause death from suffocation.

Clinical features

- Ingestion of corrosive acids causes oral pain, dysphagia, drooling, and pain in the throat, chest or abdomen. Esophageal or gastric perforation may occur.
- Cardiovascular collapse may develop soon after severe poisoning.

- Shock with cold clammy skin, weak and rapid pulse, and shallow respiration can occur with exposure to strong mineral acids.
- GI bleeding or perforation occurs acutely after grade III burns.
- Metabolic acidosis, shock, GI hemorrhage and renal failure are rare.
- Concentrated acetic or sulphuric acid exposure may cause hemolysis.
- Disseminated intravascular coagulation may be a rare complication in severe cases.
- Inhalation of corrosive fumes may cause upper respiratory tract injury, with stridor, hoarseness, wheezing and noncardiogenic pulmonary edema. In severe cases, adult respiratory distress syndrome may develop.
- Ocular exposure effects range from corneal burns to opacification, blindness. Conjunctivitis and lacrimation are common.
- Dermal toxicity ranges from irritation to full thickness burns.

Diagnosis

Diagnosis is based on history of exposure to a corrosive agent and characteristic findings. The victim complains of pain in throat due to oral burns.

Laboratory/Monitoring

- Obtain baseline CBC and electrolytes in patients with significant burns.
- Monitor renal functions and coagulation profile in patients with severe burns.
- Obtain an upright chest X-ray in patients with pulmonary symptoms or suspected perforation.

Management

Pre-hospital

- Do not induce emesis.
- Do not attempt neutralization with a basic solution and avoid carbonated beverages.
- Dilute with milk or water (120–240 ml) avoiding excessive amounts.
- Irrigate mouth with water.
- Wash affected skin with water and irrigate exposed eyes with copious amounts of water.
- Move patients of inhalation exposure to fresh air.

Hospital

- Administer oxygen to all patients with pulmonary symptoms.
- Do not perform gastric lavage because of the potential for perforation.
- Attempt suction through a soft nasogastric tube in substantial ingestion.

- Do not administer activated charcoal unless a toxic coingestant is involved.
- Administer IV fluids and vasopressors if required.
- Perform endoscopy within first 24 hrs. to predict early hemorrhage or perforation and late risk of stricture.
- Obtain chest X-ray for mediastinitis or GI perforation.
- Perform laparotomy, in case endoscopy reveals Grade III burns with thickness necrosis of esophagus or stomach or when signs and symptoms of GI perforation are evident at the time of initial presentation.
- Give antibiotics only for suspected infection or perforation.
- Role of corticosteroids is controversial.
- In case of hydrofluoric acid (HF) poisoning, monitor ECG, Ca^{2+} and K^+. If there is evidence of hypocalcemia or severe hyperkalemia, give calcium gluconate. For topical exposure apply gel containing calcium gluconate.
- In case of picric acid ingestion, administer large amounts of IV dextrose as it aids in reduction of picric acid to less poisonous picramic acid.
- In case of formic acid ingestion, correct metabolic acidosis with sodium bicarbonate.
- Hemodialysis is effective in formic acid ingestion.
- There is no specific antidote for most of the agents.

Alkalies

Caustic alkaline substances include ammonia, calcium carbide, calcium hydroxide, calcium oxide, caustic potash, caustic soda (sodium hydroxide), clinitest tablets, potassium carbonate, sodium carbonate, trisodium phosphate etc. Ammonia is a highly volatile and water soluble alkali. Anhydrous ammonia is a colourless, irritating, noxious, water soluble gas used in the manufacture of fertilizers, plastics, explosives, nylon and as a commercial refrigerant gas. Household ammonia solutions are 5–10% aqueous solutions. Solutions greater than 10% are corrosive. Ingestion of industrial strength, 30% or greater, can produce strictures. Aqueous ammonia and chlorine bleach produce chloramine gas which causes pulmonary injury. Calcium oxide (lime) when mixed with water forms calcium hydroxide. Dry calcium hydroxide is corrosive and a strong irritant (pH 11–13) used in making Portland cement. Potassium hydroxide (KOH) or caustic potash less than 1% is a weak irritant, and solutions of greater than 1% are corrosive. Potassium permanganate ($KMnO_4$) is an oxidizer with corrosive properties.

Alkaline corrosives are used as drain openers, oven cleaners, dairy and industrial pipeline cleaners, bathroom and household cleaners, hair relaxers (pH 11–14), cleaners of non-disposable glass containers, electric dishwasher soaps and low phosphate detergents. Clinitest tablets contain sodium hydroxide (50%), sodium carbonate, copper sulphate and citric acid producing corrosive burns when swallowed. Trisodium phosphate, silicates and carbonates (laundry and automatic dishwasher detergents) are caustic in nature. Household bleaches (4–6% sodium hypochlorite) are capable of producing superficial mucosal burns.

Mechanism of toxicity

Alkaline corrosives cause liquefactive necrosis, allowing deep penetration into mucosal tissue as cells are destroyed. Concentrated solutions can produce transmural necrosis with exposures as short as one second. Solid agents produce the greatest damage in the mouth, pharynx and upper esophagus, while gastric damage from liquid alkalies is more extensive.

Toxic dose

Just a few milliliters of highly caustic alkali (sodium hydroxide) can cause severe injury. The toxic doses of other alkalies vary widely.

Clinical features

- Ingestion may produce burns in the oropharynx, upper airway, esophagus, and occasionally stomach. Absence of visible oral burns does not reliably exclude the presence of esophageal burns. Presence of stridor, vomiting and drooling are associated with serious esophageal injury in most cases.
- Metabolic acidosis may develop in patients with severe GI bleeding or massive tissue necrosis after ingestion of corrosive agents.
- Renal failure is a rare complication of severe burns, accompanied by shock and GI bleeding.
- Inhalation of alkaline vapours may cause upper airway edema, respiratory failure, wheezing, pulmonary edema, and pneumonitis.
- Ocular exposure may produce severe conjunctival irritation and chemosis, corneal epithelial defects, limbal ischemia, permanent visual loss and perforation in severe cases.
- Dermal contact with alkaline corrosives may produce pain, redness, irritation or full thickness burns of skin.

Diagnosis

Diagnosis is based on history of exposure and pH of the substance.

Laboratory/Monitoring

- Obtain CBC in patients symptomatic of alkaline corrosive ingestion.
- Obtain renal function tests, PT or INR, PTT, type and cross match for blood in severe burns, perforation or bleeding.
- Obtain chest X-ray.

Management

Pre-hospital

- Dilute immediately with milk or water, avoiding excessive amounts.
- Do not induce emesis.
- Do not administer activated charcoal unless a coingestant is suspected.
- Irrigate exposed eyes with sterile water or saline for at least 20 min. and continue until the pH returns to normal.

Hospital

- Provide supportive and symptomatic care.
- Ensure clear airway and provide ventilatory support if required.
- Administer IV fluids and vasopressors if required.
- Avoid prophylactic use of antibiotics.
- Steroids may be tried in patients with Grade II burns.
- Surgical evaluation must be considered for any patient with Grade III esophageal injury.
- There is no specific antidote for alkaline corrosive poisoning.

Bleaches

Household bleaches commonly contain sodium hypochlorite in low concentrations (8%). Industrial and commercial products contain hypochlorite in concentrations more than 10%. Other substances used as bleaches in home include hydrogen peroxide, borate and oxalic acid in different concentrations and pH, and may produce toxicity.

Sodium hypochlorite

Sodium hypochlorite is a white, crystalline solid. The aqueous solution is greenish yellow in colour with a characteristic odour. Sodium hypochlorite is usually found as 5.4% solution in household bleaches for use in washing machines and other clean up procedures.

Mechanism of toxicity

Sodium hypochlorite upon contact with mucous membranes produces hypochlorous acid which is an irritant and may be corrosive.

Toxic dose

Exposure to liquid household bleaches rarely results in caustic injury, however caustic injury is caused following ingestion of large amounts (≥ 5 ml/kg).

Clinical features

- Hypochlorite bleaches rarely produce esophageal burns.

- Ingestion causes difficulty in swallowing, drooling, burns in mouth or oropharynx, pain in mouth, throat, chest or abdomen.
- Strictures or perforation is unlikely.
- High concentrations may cause hypotension, bradycardia, and cardiac arrest.
- Massive ingestions may produce hyperchloremic metabolic acidosis.

Diagnosis

Diagnosis is based on history of exposure and characteristic odour, accompanied by irritating or corrosive effects on the eyes, skin, or upper respiratory or GI tract.

Laboratory/Monitoring

- Monitor electrolytes in patients with large ingestions of sodium hypochlorite.
- Monitor pulse oximetry or arterial blood gases.
- Chest X-ray and pulmonary function tests are indicated in patients with significant pulmonary signs or symptoms.

Management

Pre-hospital

- Do not induce emesis.
- Dilute immediately with water or milk (120–240 ml) avoiding excessive amounts.
- Remove contaminated clothing in case of dermal exposure and wash skin with lots of water.
- Irrigate eyes gently with water for atleast 15 min. in case of ocular exposure.
- In case of inhalation exposure, if cough and respiratory distress fail to respond to fresh air within a few minutes to an hour then shift the patient immediately to a hospital.

Hospital

- Provide symptomatic and supportive care.
- Do not perform gastric lavage.
- Perform endoscopy to evaluate serious esophageal or gastric injury.
- Obtain chest and abdominal X-rays to look for GI perforation.
- Use bronchodilators for wheezing and treat non-cardiogenic pulmonary edema.
- There is no specific antidote.

Hydrogen peroxide

Hydrogen peroxide (H_2O_2) is a colourless liquid with a bitter taste. It releases oxygen bubbles on contact with tissues. Synonyms of hydrogen peroxide include carbamide peroxide, hydrogen dioxide, peroxide etc.

Hydrogen peroxide is marketed as aqueous solution of concentrations ranging from 3–90% by weight. Most industrial applications utilize concentrations varying from 35% to 70% by weight. It is commonly used as a topical antiseptic, household cleanser, in plastic manufacturing, printing, bleaching, refining oils and fats, dyes, photography, cleaning metals and as an oxidizer and disinfectant.

Mechanism of toxicity

The toxicity of H_2O_2 results from its interaction with catalase in tissues liberating water and oxygen upon decomposition. One milliliter of 3% H_2O_2 liberates 10ml of oxygen.

Toxic dose

Hydrogen peroxide (3%) is a local irritant. Higher concentrations (35%) can cause severe tissue injury and burns. A few ounces (several gulps) of hydrogen peroxide in concentrations greater than 35% has resulted in widespread gas embolization and death in both adults and children.

Clinical features

- No significant features occur after ingestion of a dilute solution as it is converted into water and oxygen in the stomach.
- Moderate ingestion may cause gastric distention and rarely perforation. Corrosive injury and air embolus have also been reported (>10%).
- Coma, cyanosis, hypotension, heart block, metabolic acidosis and seizures develop if ingested in high concentrations or in large amounts.
- Uncommon features include severe hemorrhagic gastritis and marked cerebral edema, which may lead to herniation.

Diagnosis

Diagnosis is based on history of exposure and clinical features.

Laboratory/Monitoring

- Monitor arterial blood gases and ECG in patients with suspected embolization.
- Obtain abdominal X-ray.
- Perform endoscopy in patients with ingestions of ≥ 10% solutions.

Management

Pre-hospital

- Dilute immediately with water or milk.
- Do not induce emesis.

Hospital

- Provide supportive and symptomatic care.
- Ensure clear airway and provide ventilatory support if necessary.
- Perform gastric lavage cautiously.
- Activated charcoal and cathartics are not effective.
- There is no specific antidote.

Boric acid and Borates

Borates exist in both alkaline and acidic forms. Sodium borate (borax) is an alkaline salt which is used as an antiseptic and cleansing agent. Borax cleaners contain 21.5% boron by dry weight.

Boric acid is found as colourless and odourless crystals, granules or white powder. Powdered boric acid (99%) is still used as a pesticide against ants and cockroaches. It is used as an antiseptic, disinfectant, astringent, food preservative, water softener, mild antiseptic eyewash (5%, 10%) and optic solution (5%) and a fungistatic agent in baby talcum powder.

Mechanism of toxicity

The mechanism of borate poisoning is unknown. Boric acid is not highly corrosive. It probably acts as a generalized cellular poison. Organ systems most commonly affected are the GIT, brain, liver and kidneys. Boric acid is well absorbed from GIT, open wounds, inflamed and denuded skin, and serous cavities.

Toxic dose

The acute oral toxic dose of boric acid is highly variable, but serious poisoning is reported to occur with the ingestion of 1–3 g of it in neonates, 5 g in infants, and 20 g in adults. Chronic ingestion or application to abraded skin is much more serious than acute single ingestion.

Clinical features

- Acute boric acid ingestion causes gastroenteritis with blue green vomitus and diarrhea. Sometimes stools become black.
- CNS stimulation may be produced.
- In severe cases, seizures and coma can occur.
- Renal failure may develop.

Diagnosis

Diagnosis is based on history of exposure, presence of gastroenteritis (possibly with blue-green vomitus), erythrodermic rash and elevated serum borate levels.

Laboratory/Monitoring

- Blood borate levels may be useful to establish the diagnosis and course of therapy.
- Monitor renal function tests, cardiovascular status, fluid and electrolyte balance in symptomatic patients.

Management

Pre-hospital

- Induce emesis with syrup of ipecac.
- Administer activated charcoal.

Hospital

- Treatment is supportive and symptomatic.
- Administer IV fluids and vasopressors if required.
- Treat coma, seizures, hypotension and renal failure if they occur.
- Hemodialysis, peritoneal dialysis and exchange transfusion may enhance elimination.
- There is no specific antidote.

Detergents and Soaps

Detergents are synthetic surface-active agents chemically classified into anionic, nonionic or cationic groups. Bleaching (chlorine-releasing), bacteriostatic (low concentration of quaternary ammonium compounds) or enzymatic agents are found in most products. They are non-soap surfactants in combination with inorganic ingredients (phosphates, silicates and carbonates). Soaps are salts of fatty acids and are of low toxicity.

Household detergents usually contain anionic or nonionic surfactants while cationic and amphoteric surfactants are used in laundries. The anionic laundry detergents are alkyl sodium sulphates, alkylbenzene sulphonates and sodium lauryl sulphate. Dish washer detergents are polyoxyethylene alkyl ethers also called ethoxylated alcohols (nonionic). Many detergents contain inorganic salts as "builders" or water softeners to enhance function in hard water. The inorganic ingredient of a detergent maintains the proper pH and combines with calcium and other minerals in hard water that interfere with cleaning. Cationic detergents are quaternary ammonium compounds such as benzalkonium chloride, benzethonium chloride, alkyl dimethyl-3,

4-dichlorobenzene ammonium chloride. Fabric softeners also contain cationic detergents.

Mechanism of toxicity

Detergents and soaps are irritants and toxicity is generally limited to cutaneous, ocular, oral or GI irritation. They may precipitate and denature proteins, are irritating to tissues and possess keratolytic and corrosive action. Anionic and nonionic detergents are only mildly irritating, but cationic detergents are more hazardous because quaternary ammonium compounds are caustic.

Toxic dose

Mortality and serious morbidity are rare. Cationic and dishwasher detergents are more dangerous than anionic and nonionic products. The estimated toxic dose of cationic detergents is 30 mg/kg and the potentially fatal dose is 1 to 3 g.

Clinical features

- Immediate spontaneous emesis often occurs after oral ingestion. Large ingestion may produce intractable vomiting, diarrhea and hematemesis.
- Aspiration may result in upper airway edema and significant respiratory distress.
- Low phosphate detergents are generally more alkaline and ingestion may result in oral and esophageal burns. They may produce hypocalcemia and tetany.
- Cationic surfactants are more toxic than anionic or nonionic surfactants and their concentrated solutions act like corrosives.
- Systemic absorption of cationic surfactants may produce restlessness, confusion, convulsions, respiratory paralysis, muscle weakness and cyanosis.
- Dishwashing detergents have a higher pH due to the addition of alkaline builders and may produce serious injury to exposed tissues.
- Eye exposure may cause mild to serious corrosive injury depending upon the specific product.
- Dermal contact generally causes a mild erythema or rash.

Diagnosis

Diagnosis is based on history of exposure and prompt onset of vomiting. Frothing mouth may also suggest exposure.

Laboratory/Monitoring

- Monitor fluid status and electrolytes in patients with persistent vomiting or diarrhea.
- If respiratory tract irritation or respiratory depression is evident, monitor arterial blood gases, chest X-ray and pulmonary function tests.

Management

Pre-hospital

- Emesis rarely needs to be induced as detergents themselves have emetic properties.
- Immediately dilute with milk or water in adults (120–240 ml, not to exceed 15 ml/kg in a child).
- Irrigate eyes with copious amounts of tepid water or saline and seek advice of ophthalmologist if eye pain persists.
- Wash affected skin with copious amounts of water.

Hospital

- Ingestion of nonionic or anionic detergents is generally self limiting, requiring no treatment.
- Provide ventilatory support if required.
- Maintain fluid and electrolyte balance if excessive vomiting or diarrhea occurs.
- Manage as for corrosive ingestion if a highly alkaline detergent or bleach is ingested.
- Observe for the possible development of esophageal or GI irritation or burns.
- If corrosive injury is suspected, consult a gastroenterologist for possible endoscopy.
- Administer methylene blue in case of methemoglobinemia.
- If symptomatic hypocalcemia occurs after ingestion of a phosphate-containing product, administer IV calcium.

Antiseptics

Dettol
Dettol is the most common household antiseptic and disinfectant. Accidental ingestion by children is not uncommon as it is often within their reach. Dettol is a mixture of approximately 4.8% chloroxylenol, pine oil, isopropyl alcohol and possibly castor oil and soap. It has also been used as a substance of abuse, and ingested in suicide attempts.

Mechanism of toxicity
Chloroxylenol is mainly effective against gram positive bacteria, however it is less active against *Staphylococci* and gram negative bacteria, and ineffective against *Pseudomonas* and bacterial spores.

Toxic dose
Toxicity has resulted after ingestion of 20–600 ml in an adult and 120 ml in

a child. Death or severe morbidity has been attributed to aspiration during gastric lavage.

Clinical features

- Ingestion leads to sore throat, burns of the buccal cavity, vomiting and tachycardia.
- CNS depression ranges from drowsiness to coma.
- Injury to the larynx can result in airway obstruction, aspiration with secondary symptoms of adult respiratory distress syndrome (ARDS) or pneumonia and hypotension.
- Shock and hypothermia may be observed.
- ECG may reveal non-specific ST-T changes.
- Renal effects are reported after large ingestions (200–500 ml).
- Allergic contact dermatitis is noted after dermal exposure.

Diagnosis

Diagnosis is based on history of exposure and/or hoarseness, dysphagia, soreness and erythema of the mouth and throat that occur frequently after ingestion.

Laboratory/Monitoring

- Monitor electrolytes, liver function tests, BUN, creatinine and CPK.
- Obtain chest X-ray to evaluate possible pulmonary aspiration and secondary effects.

Management

Pre-hospital

- Do not induce emesis.
- Dilution is controversial as it may increase the risk of vomiting and aspiration. However, consider only if the patient is conscious and fully alert.
- Use of activated charcoal is controversial.
- Wash exposed skin with lots of water.
- Irrigate eyes with copious amounts of water.

Hospital

- Treatment is supportive and symptomatic.
- Support respiratory and cardiovascular functions.
- Perform gastric lavage.
- Treat hypotension with IV fluids and vasopressors if required.
- Monitor respiratory status carefully and frequently for several hours for the development of laryngeal edema, airway constriction and respiratory distress.

- Observe patients of inhalation exposure carefully for the development of systemic signs and symptoms and provide symptomatic treatment as necessary.
- There is no specific antidote.

Savlon

Savlon, a general topical antiseptic, contains chlorhexidine. It is a cationic biguanide compound also used in mouthwashes. Liquid savlon contains chlorhexidine gluconate (1.5%) and cetrimide (3%). Savlon/cetavlex cream has chlorhexidine HCl (0.1%) and cetrimide (0.5%) while savlon hospital concentrate contains chlorhexidine gluconate (7.5%) and cetrimide (15%).

Mechanism of toxicity

Chlorhexidine is a protein denaturant. It is a powerful non-irritating antiseptic that disrupts bacterial cell membrane. It is relatively more active against gram positive bacteria and like hexachlorophene, persists on skin.

Toxic dose

Toxicity is primarily related to irritant or caustic effect, depending on concentration. Ingestion of 4% solution is expected to be irritating. Hepatotoxicity in adults is reported with ingestion of 400 mg/kg .

Clinical features

- Ingestion of large amount of a concentrated solution (20%) may result in esophageal necrosis and hepatotoxicity. Little systemic absorption occurs, thus the primary expected effect is irritation in lower concentrations and corrosive effects in higher concentrations.
- Eye exposure to a 4% solution may cause reversible corneal injury.

Diagnosis

Diagnosis is based on history of exposure and the presence of a characteristic odour.

Laboratory/Monitoring

- Monitor liver function tests in patients with substantial ingestions.

Management

Pre-hospital

- Do not induce emesis. Emesis may be spontaneous with products containing anionic surfactants or isopropyl alcohol.

Hospital

- Treatment is supportive and symptomatic.

- Dilute with water for small ingestions.
- Consider gastric lavage for very large amounts.
- There is no specific antidote.

Iodine

The chief use of iodine is because of its antiseptic property. It is poorly soluble in water and liquid formulations are usually prepared and marketed as a tincture in ethanol (50% or higher). Typically, the tincture and other solutions contain potassium or sodium salts which enhance solubility. It is widely used as an antiseptic, germicide and water treatment chemical. It is used in dyes, X-ray media and photographic chemicals. It is most commonly used as the USP tincture (2% iodine + 2% sodium iodide in 50% alcohol, 5 ml = 100 mg iodine). Other iodine formulations official in IP are strong iodine tincture (7% iodine + 5% potassium iodide in 83% alcohol, 5 ml = 350 mg iodine), Lugol's solution (5% iodine + 10% potassium iodide in aqueous solution) and iodine ointment (4% iodine). The iodine salt in these solutions does not contribute to the toxicity of these agents. Povidone-iodine is a commonly available iodophor disinfectant. Iodinated glycerol is used as an expectorant.

Mechanism of toxicity

Iodine is corrosive because of its oxidizing properties. When ingested, it is poorly absorbed but may cause severe gastroenteritis. It is readily inactivated by starch and converted to iodide, which is non toxic. In the body, iodine is rapidly converted to iodide and stored in the thyroid gland.

Toxic dose

The toxic dose depends on the product and the route of exposure. Iodophors and iodoform liberate only small amounts of iodine and are generally nontoxic and non caustic. Ingestion of 4 g of iodine and 40 ml of iodine tincture are reported to be fatal in children and adults respectively.

Clinical features

- Ingestion can cause corrosive gastroenteritis with vomiting, hematemesis and diarrhea, resulting in significant volume loss and circulatory collapse.
- Mucous membranes are usually stained brown, and the vomitus may be blue if starchy foods are already present in the stomach.
- Pharyngeal swelling and glottic edema have been reported.
- Inhalation of iodine vapours can cause severe pulmonary irritation leading to pulmonary edema.
- Skin and eye exposures may result in severe corrosive burns.
- Skin exposure to strong iodine tincture may cause dermal necrosis.

Diagnosis

Diagnosis is based on history of exposure and evidence of corrosive injury. Mucous membranes are usually stained brown and vomitus may be blue.

Laboratory/Monitoring

- Plasma iodine levels are not clinically useful but may aid in diagnosis.
- Monitor fluid and electrolyte status carefully in severely symptomatic patients.
- Monitor CBC.
- Monitor renal function tests and urinalysis in patients with significant exposure.
- Monitor arterial blood gases or oximetry. Obtain chest X-ray in serious inhalation exposure.

Management

Pre-hospital

- Remove victim to fresh air after inhalation exposure.
- Irrigate exposed eyes with tepid water or saline for atleast 15 minutes.
- Wash skin with copious amounts of water.
- Do not induce emesis.
- Administer a starchy food (potato, flour, cornstarch) or milk to lessen GI irritation.

Hospital

- Provide supportive treatment.
- Maintain airway and perform endotracheal intubation if airway edema is progressive.
- For large exposures, consider gastric lavage using milk or corn starch.
- Treat bronchospasm and pulmonary edema if they occur.
- Administer IV fluids.
- In case of corrosive injury to the esophagus or stomach, perform endoscopy.
- Sodium thiosulphate may convert iodine to iodide and tetrathionate, but is not recommended for intravenous use because iodine is rapidly converted to iodide in the body.

6. Miscellaneous Household Products

Button batteries

Button batteries are available in a variety of sizes and chemical systems and are intended for use in hearing aids, watches, calculators, photographic equipments, toys, game articles, remote control devices and musical greeting cards. Commonly ingested chemical systems include mercuric oxide, silver oxide, manganese dioxide and zinc air cells, all of which contain an alkaline electrolyte (26–45% sodium or potassium hydroxide). They contain metal oxide and dioxide cathodes and zinc anodes. Zinc air cells used predominantly in hearing aids are air-activated upon removal of seal and recognized readily by the presence of several pores through the battery which allow air entry. An alkaline electrolyte which is the only potentially hazardous ingredient is enclosed behind a membrane through which the air penetrates. Lithium batteries are used in pacemakers. Most of the ingested button batteries negotiate the gastrointestinal tract uneventfully but passage may require upto 14 days. Though complications after ingestion are rare, batteries lodged predominantly in the esophagus may be associated with severe complications. Button batteries in the stomach are usually asymptomatic. Though mercury batteries tend to open, clinical toxicity is unlikely because mercuric oxide is converted to the considerably less toxic and poorly absorbed elemental mercury as the battery discharges. In addition, mercuric oxide which leaks and slowly solubilizes, is formed in a compacted amalgam and may also be reduced in the stomach to elemental mercury through chemical reaction with iron released from the corroding battery can.

Mechanism of toxicity
Button batteries cause tissue injury by actual leakage of alkaline electrolyte from within the battery leading to localized tissue necrosis and local tissue damage by the electrical current generated external to the battery. In addition to the direct injury by the electrical current, clinically significant local concentrations of sodium hydroxide may be generated due to electrolysis of sodium chloride within the tissue causing subsequent injury even in the absence of actual cell leakage. Further, constant pressure by the impacted battery on the adjacent tissue may also lead to tissue necrosis.

Clinical features

- Esophageal battery lodgement occurs with ingestion of batteries larger than 23.0 mm diameter. It can occur with smaller batteries also in very young children. Disc batteries with less than 15.6 mm diameter do not get lodged in esophagus.
- Esophageal burns are noted within 4 hrs. of ingestion.
- Early manifestations include irritability, pain or discomfort on swallowing, fever, vomiting and refusal to take food.
- Esophageal perforation, mediastinitis with multiple complications like tracheo esophageal fistula and pneumothorax may occur.
- Majority of batteries pass through the GIT without complications if esophageal impaction does not occur.
- Significant morbidity is uncommon once the battery passes beyond esophagus.
- Rarely it can get lodged in Meckel's diverticulum.
- Severe local tissue injury and erosions through the external ear canal occur when placed in the ear.
- Nasal septal perforations, erosions into the mastoid cavity and severe local tissue injury may occur when a battery is placed in the nose.

Diagnosis

It is based on history of ingestion. X-ray localization is recommended in all cases of suspected button battery ingestion to confirm the diagnosis. Disc batteries are differentiated from foreign bodies like coins by their typical double contour.

Laboratory/Monitoring

- Take initial chest and abdomen X-rays to determine the location of the ingested battery and follow by subsequent radiographs to see its progress through the GIT.
- If mercury exposure is suspected, obtain blood and urinary mercury concentrations.

Management

Prehospital

- Do not induce emesis.
- Do not give activated charcoal.

Hospital

- Follow initial radiographs by subsequent ones.
- Take X-ray from nasopharynx down to the rectal areas including both a PA and lateral film.

- Hospitalization may not be required if the battery has passed beyond esophagus, Patients should watch out for vomiting, tarry or bloody stools, fever, abdominal pain or decreased appetite.
- Perform a repeat X-ray in the absence of symptoms, 4 to 7 days after the ingestion if the battery passage in the stool is not documented. In case of associated symptoms with battery transit arrest, endoscopic or surgical intervention is indicated.
- Remove batteries located in the esophagus immediately by endoscopy.
- Remove a badly corroding battery by endoscopy or surgery. Such a removal is considered when the battery stops progressing through the GIT.
- Administration of cathartics, metoclopramide, cimetidine has not been found to be effective.
- Laparotomy is indicated in case of a failure in endoscopic removal in a symptomatic patient, mucosal damage or a badly corroding battery and in case there are signs of peritonitis or when less invasive techniques fail to retrieve the battery in an asymptomatic patient.
- In case button cell is split on X-ray, especially, where visible droplet like opacities are noted on abdominal X-ray (possibly a mercuric oxide chemical system), remove the split battery promptly by purging or enema and check urinary and blood mercury levels.
- For batteries in ear or nose, remove them promptly avoiding nasal or optic drops before removal and also avoid alligator forceps and biting instruments. Irrigate the site thoroughly with water to remove remaining foreign material.

Thermometers

Clinical thermometers contain elemental mercury which is absorbed poorly from the gastrointestinal tract. Acute ingestion has caused poisoning only in presence of abnormal gut motility that markedly delays fecal elimination. Elemental mercury ingestion does not require any specific treatment.

Typewriter correction fluids

The general formulations contain trichloroethylene, trichloroethane and inert pigments. Inhalation abuse of typewriter correction fluid containing trichloroethylene has been reported, however, most brands no longer contain it now. The predominant physiologic response is CNS depression. Trichloroethane is a CNS and respiratory depressant as well as skin and mucous membrane irritant. Recreational abuse may produce unconsciousness, seizures, respiratory arrest, dysrhythmias and sudden death. Treatment is supportive.

Matches

The general formulations of "strike anywhere" or kitchen match head contain potassium chlorate, phosphorous sesquisulfide, glue, sulphur, powdered glass, resins and dyes. The stick contains paraffin and ammonium phosphate in traces. The striking surface contains silica flour and usually red phosphorous, both being non toxic. Chlorates are very potent oxidising agents and exposure may result in GI symptoms, hemolysis with methemoglobin formation and renal failure. The heads of less than twenty large matches contain approximately 330 mg and twenty small heads contain 220 mg of potassium chlorate which is not enough to be harmful to a child. An acute or cumulative dose of 7.5–35 g has been shown to be lethal in adults. Thus toxicity is unlikely even after ingestion of several match sticks. The treatment is symptomatic. Sodium thiosulphate can be given orally or intravenously to inactivate the chlorate ion to less toxic chloride ions. Methemoglobinemia may be unresponsive to methylene blue and ascorbic acid. Diuretics may be needed to maintain diuresis. Exchange transfusion combined with hemodialysis has been the most successful treatment in severe poisoning.

Shaving creams

The general composition of shaving creams is soap, perfume, menthol and antiseptics. Aerosol, brushless and lather shaving creams contain fatty acid alcohol and amine soaps, humectants, essential oil (fragrance) emulsifiers and a propellant. However, the concentrations vary in different formulations. Gastrointestinal symptoms are likely only after a substantial ingestion, which is usually unlikely. The treatment is supportive and symptomatic in case of development of any clinical features.

Deodorants

Antiperspirants contain ethyl alcohol, antiperspirant salts like aluminium chlorhydroxide, deodorants, oils, humectants, suspending agents and a propellant. The primary effects caused by exposure to antiperspirants include skin and eye irritation, gastrointestinal irritation and contact dermatitis. A transient cough may occur following inhalation exposure. Ingestion of deodorants may require dilution with water or milk. No specific treatment is indicated.

Shampoos

Shampoos contain anionic, nonionic and amphoteric surfactants, preservatives, colouring agents, thickners and humectants. Ingestion is unlikely to cause any systemic effect unless large quantities are consumed. Gastric irritation may be managed with milk or water and or with H_2 blockers.

Aftershave lotions

The general formulations of aftershave lotions and colognes contain ethanol in varying amounts (50–90%) and perfumes. Ingestion may cause dizziness and hypoglycemia. Treatment is supportive and symptomatic.

Skin lotions and creams

They generally contain laxatives, wax, fat or oil, humectants, water, thickeners, colouring agents, fragrance, preservatives and ethanol (10% or less). Toxicity following acute ingestion of excessive amounts is generally minimal and limited to gastrointestinal tract and the management of symptoms if any, is supportive and symptomatic.

Nail polishes

Nail polishes usually contain solvents (toluene, xylene, acetone, ethanol, isopropyl alcohol, ethyl, butyl or amyl acetates), plasticizers, cellulose acetate or nitrocellulose, resins, dyes and pearling agents. Ingestion of large amounts may cause nausea, vomiting and CNS depression (narcosis). Symptoms of methanol and aromatic hydrocarbon poisoning may also precipitate. In small ingestions (20 ml), dilution with milk or water is advisable.

Nail polish removers

Nail polish removers contain solvents (acetone, ethanol, isopropyl alcohol, methanol, ethyl and butyl acetate), mineral spirits, emollients and fragrance. Toxicity is due to the solvents. Ingestion of large amounts may precipitate symptoms of solvent poisoning. Small amount ingestion is managed with water or milk.

Hair bleaches

Hair bleaches usually consist of two parts, the bleach base which contains fats, oils, gels, nonionic surfactants and humectants, ammonia and ammonium persulphate and the other part consisting of hydrogen peroxide. Moderate toxicity results due to ingestion. However, due to gritty sensation in the mouth and disagreeable taste, ingestion of significant amounts is unlikely. Ingestion is managed by irrigating mouth with water and dilution with milk.

Lipsticks

Lipsticks contain oils like castor oil, wax, perfume, antioxidants and preservatives, lanolin, colouring agents, pearling agents (bismuth oxychloride). Lipstick ingestion is considered non toxic.

Perfumes

The general formulation of perfumes comprises of ethanol (75–95%) and essential oil (5–25%). In addition, water, traces of colour and propellants may also be present. Ingestion may cause dizziness and hypoglycemia especially in children. Perfumes cause local irritation in eyes. Management is supportive.

Talc

Talc powders contain talc, calcium or magnesium carbonate, zinc stearate, kaolin, perfume and preservatives. Ingestion is generally non toxic. Acute inhalation may result in difficult breathing, respiratory distress and sometimes death due to asphyxia.

Hair dyes

Hair dyes may impart temporary or permanent colour to the hair. The temporary hair dyes usually contain fatty acid alcohols, quaternary detergents, coconut or other fatty acids, alkonalamines and esters, propylene glycol, isopropanol, aromatic and nitrosamine compounds. The permanent dyes usually contain a developer (6% solution of hydrogen peroxide) as an oxidising agent and various dye intermediates like p-phenylenediamine, substituted phenylenediamines, amino phenols, resorcinol, catechol and pyrogallol in a base which is an aqueous solution of soap. Paraphenylenediamine gives a brown or black shade to hair. Its typical concentrations range from 0.2% in blonde dyes to 4% in black dyes. Toxic effects are not observed following ingestion of significant amounts usually due to reflex vomiting because the developer may contain free ammonia. Furthermore, in formulations where hydrogen peroxide is used, acute oral toxicity is minimal due to its low concentration. Mouth irrigation and administration of milk is helpful for any oral or gastric irritation. Eye or skin exposure may cause mild irritation which is resolved by washing with water.

Holi colours

The commonly available colours used in the festival of Holi mainly contain colours, crushed glass, mica, corrosives and sand. The colours used are either water colours, dry powders or pastes. Sometimes they are mixed with oil for application. Dry colour powders (gulals) contain heavy metals like cadmium, chromium, iron, nickel, mercury, lead, zinc etc in a silica or asbestos base. All these heavy metals are documented to be systemic toxins whereas silica and asbestos may cause dermal manifestations like irritation, itching, redness, abrasions etc. Further, respiratory symptoms are also noted with dry powders. Among the water colours, gentian violet is commonly used. Its concentrated solutions can cause dermatitis, skin allergy and irritation of mucous membranes. Keratoconjunctivitis and staining of cornea is also reported. Many other water colours have an alkaline base which can cause corrosive burns on skin or after eye contact. The colour pastes imparting different colours contain highly toxic metal salts like aluminium bromide (silver), mercury sulphite (red), copper sulphate (blue) and lead oxide (black). These mainly cause dermatological and ocular effects.

The management of toxicity is supportive and symptomatic. The affected skin should be washed thoroughly with copious amounts of soap and water and eyes irrigated with tepid water for at least 15 minutes. Dermatological and ophthalmological consultations should be taken in case of any complication. All Holi colours should be used with caution as some of them are carcinogenic.

Parad

Parad is commonly used in households as a preservative for rice. It contains elemental mercury as the main ingredient. Toxicity is expected only after substantial acute ingestion. There is minimal absorption through GIT in healthy individuals. Ingestion of extremely large amounts or in patients with abnormally diminished bowel motility or intestinal perforation, there is a risk of toxicity. Fecal excretion helps in its elimination. Patients usually do not present with any symptoms. However, in substantial ingestion the management includes gastric lavage and multiple dose cathartics with a proper watch on electrolyte balance. No chelation therapy is required in acute ingestion.

Non toxic ingestions

These mainly include pencil lead, crayons, silica gel, oral contraceptives, glues, teething rings, unsmoked cigarettes filter tips, erasers, air freshners etc.

7. Industrial Chemicals

Copper sulphate

Copper sulphate is a blue, crystalline or granular powder. Its anhydrous form is white in colour. It is used as a fungicide, algicide, herbicide, molluscide and also in steel and petroleum industry.

Mechanism of toxicity
Copper inhibits enzymes G-6-PD and glutathione reductase which are important in protecting the cell from oxygen free radicals. Lipid peroxidation and significant increase of copper content in the mitochondrion suggest hepatic mitochondrion to be an important target in hepatic toxicity, with an involvement of oxidant damage to the liver. Hemolysis is produced by increasing oxidation of hemoglobin sulfhydryl groups, leading to increased red blood cell permeability.

Toxic dose
Ingestion of 250 mg can cause toxicity and 10–20 mg is lethal. The lowest oral toxic dose reported is 120 µg/kg. Serum copper levels above 500µg/dl are associated with severe toxicity (normal range 89–137 µg/dl in males and 87–153 µg/dl in females). Whole blood copper concentration of 3 mg/L is associated with toxicity. Severe hepatic disorder has been reported in children after ingestion of 10mg of copper in contaminated milk. Inhalation of 60–100 mg/kg of copper dust produces gastrointestinal effects.

Clinical features
- Ingestion causes abdominal pain, nausea, vomiting, diarrhea, salivation and metallic taste.
- Stools, vomitus, saliva and mucous membranes are often stained green or blue.
- Extensive corrosion and necrosis of GIT may take place.
- Jaundice due to both hemolysis as well as direct liver damage may be produced.
- Oliguria and renal failure can occur due to direct toxicity as well as intravascular hemolysis.

- Intravascular hemolysis and hemoglobinuria occur 12–24 hrs. after ingestion.
- In severe cases seizures, delirium and coma may occur.
- Methemoglobinemia may be produced.
- Hypotension and hyperthermia may occur.
- Complete paralysis of limbs is rarely observed.
- It can cause dermal irritation on contact.

Diagnosis

Diagnosis is based on history of exposure. Ingestion of copper salts results in gastroenteritis. Inhalation of copper fumes is associated with fever and respiratory complaints.

Laboratory/Monitoring

- Monitor whole blood copper levels in symptomatic patients.
- Obtain baseline liver and renal functions tests, CBC and arterial blood gases.
- Estimate methemoglobin levels in cyanotic patients.
- Obtain chest X-ray.

Management

Pre-hospital

- Dilute with water or milk.
- Do not induce emesis.
- Irrigate exposed eyes or skin with copious amounts of water.

Hospital

- Provide symptomatic and supportive care.
- Perform gastric lavage.
- Treat shock with IV fluids and vasopressors as needed.
- Consider endoscopy to assess the extent of burn injury to the GIT.
- Burn injury if any, may be treated conservatively.
- Treat methemoglobinemia with methylene blue and humidified supplemental oxygen.
- Specific antidotes are BAL and D-pencillamine which should be given to seriously ill patients with large ingestions.

Carbon monoxide

Carbon monoxide (CO) is a colourless, odourless and tasteless gas produced by the incomplete combustion of organic fuels. Exhaust fumes from internal combustion engine (automobiles and gensets), charcoal and poorly vented wood or coal stoves, kerosene lanterns, and fire in buildings are common sources of carbon monoxide poisoning. Factors that influence clinical response are age, metabolic rate, physical activity and pulmonary function or the presence of pulmonary or cardiovascular diseases.

Mechanism of toxicity

The exact mechanism of carbon monoxide poisoning is not established. It is a cellular poison, as it competes with oxygen for other hemoproteins (myoglobin, peroxidase, catalase and cytochrome). Carbon monoxide reduces the oxygen carrying capacity of hemoglobin and reduces oxygen delivery to the tissues. The affinity of carbon monoxide to bind with hemoglobin is 200 times more than that of oxygen resulting in reduced oxyhemoglobin saturation. It binds to the cytochrome oxidase system to reduce cellular utilization of oxygen. The half life of carboxyhemoglobin (COHb) is 4 hrs. when the patient breathes air, 90 min. with 100% oxygen and 30 min. with hyperbaric oxygen.

Toxic dose

Moderate toxicity is associated with an exposure level of 0.04–0.10% of CO in the atmosphere for 4 hrs. Severe toxicity is associated with an exposure level of 0.11–0.15% CO in the atmosphere for 1.5–3 hrs.

Clinical features

COHb levels of:

- 10–20% produce slight headache, exercise induced angina, or dyspnea on vigorous exertion.
- 20–30% produce throbbing headache, and dyspnea on moderate exertion.
- 30–40% produce severe headache, nausea, vomiting, weakness, dizziness, visual disturbance and impaired judgement.
- 40–50% lead to syncope, tachycardia and tachypnea.
- 50–60% produce coma, convulsions, and Cheyne-Stokes respiration.
- 60–70% result in compromised cardiorespiratory function.
- Above 60% are lethal if untreated.
- Hypotension may occur secondary to vasodilation or myocardial depression.
- Transient hypertension may occur.
- Lactic acidosis may occur.
- Hematuria, albuminuria, renal failure, myoglobinuria, and acute tubular necrosis are reported.
- Hyperglycemia may be produced.
- Survivors of severe poisoning may suffer from neurological sequelae consistent with hypoxic ischemic insult.
- Cherry red appearance of skin and mucous membranes is actually uncommon.

- Visual field deficits and retinopathy may occur.
- Severe delayed neuropathy may also be observed.

Diagnosis

There is no specific reliable clinical finding and history of exposure forms the basis of diagnosis.

Laboratory/Monitoring

- Monitor COHb levels every 4 hrs. until patient is asymptomatic or levels are within normal range.
- Monitor electrolytes, CPK, urinalysis and arterial blood gases, if patient is symptomatic or COHb levels are greater than 20%.
- Monitor cardiac functions.

Management

Pre-hospital

- Move patient to fresh air.

Hospital

- Provide symptomatic and supportive care.
- Maintain the airway and assist ventilation as required.
- Administer 100% oxygen till COHb levels are less than 5%.
- Give hyperbaric oxygen in severe cases.
- Treat hypotension with IV fluids and vasopressors (dopamine and norepinephrine in refractory cases) as needed.
- Administer anticonvulsants to control seizures. Give phenobarbital in case of recurrent seizures.

Cyanide

Cyanide is one of the most lethal chemicals available. Hydrogen cyanide is a gas produced by mixing cyanide salts with acids. It is a combustion by-product of petrochemicals, plastics, wool, silk, polyurethane bedding or furniture, acrylic baths, nylon carpets etc. and hence cyanide poisoning should be suspected in victims of smoke inhalation. Cyanide can be released by hepatic metabolism of various nitrile compounds. Alkaline cyanide salts (potassium or sodium cyanide) are used for extraction of silver or gold, recovery of metals from X-ray and photographic films, electroplating, chelation, manufacture of dyes, pigments, nylon, insecticides and fumigants. Cyanogenic glycosides are found in apple, peach, apricot, plum, cherry, cassava, cycad nut, linseed, and almond seeds. Cyanogen halides are used as warfare agents.

Mechanism of toxicity

Cyanide is a cellular poison that can readily bind to many enzymes having a metallic component. Cytochrome oxidase, the terminal enzyme involved in aerobic metabolism, is considered responsible for most of the toxic effects of cyanide. Inhibition of this enzyme results in histotoxic anoxia due to paralysis of aerobic metabolism. CNS and cardiovascular systems are susceptible to anoxia. It has been shown that cyanide initially forms a relatively stable reversible complex by binding to the protein portion of this enzyme and later gets attached to the iron component. Cyanide binds other proteins like nitrate reductase, myoglobin, ribulose diphosphate carboxylase, and catalase. Lipid metabolism and calcium transport is also altered.

Toxic dose

The fatal dose varies from 50-300mg for an adult, depending upon the agent involved. Whole blood levels above 0.5–1.0 mg/L are considered toxic.

Clinical features

- CNS effects include headache, faintness, perspiration, vertigo, anxiety/excitement, drowsiness, prostration, opisthotonos and trismus, hyperthermia, convulsions, stupor, paralysis, coma and death.
- GI effects are burning tongue, local irritation of mucous membranes, salivation, nausea and abdominal pain.
- Metabolic acidosis and elevated serum lactate levels are associated with significant exposure.
- Respiratory effects are tachypnea and dyspnea followed by slowing of respiratory rate with subsequent respiratory depression, pulmonary edema and cyanosis (late findings).
- Cardiovascular features include hypertension with reflux bradycardia, and sinus arrhythmia followed by tachycardia with hypotension and cardiovascular collapse. ECG changes include QRS complex changes, elevated T waves, shortened QT segment with eventual fusion of the T wave into the QRS complex. The heart continues to beat for several minutes even after complete depression of respiration.
- Mydriasis and red colouration of both retinal arteries and veins appear similar.
- Inhalation results in vomiting, headache, dyspnea, fatigue, confusion, seizures and coma. Circulatory collapse and death may occur within minutes.
- Dermal exposure produces irritation and pruritis. Moist sodium cyanide may cause burns.

Diagnosis

History of exposure is the basis of diagnosis. Cyanide poisoning should be suspected in victims of smoke inhalation. With cyanide poisoning the veins have a red colour in contrast to the usual blue tint and are difficult to distinguish from arteries. This is due to decreased tissue extraction of oxygen resulting in high venous oxygen saturation. Odour of bitter almonds is likely to be missed.

Laboratory/Monitoring

- Monitor for lactic acidosis.
- Obtain blood glucose, electrolytes and arterial blood gases.
- Estimate blood cyanide levels (levels greater than 2.5 μg/ml are associated with severe poisoning and levels greater than 3 μg/ml are considered to be lethal).
- Monitor ECG.

Management

Pre-hospital

- Remove the patient from the site of exposure in case of inhalation.
- Wash affected skin thoroughly with water.
- Do not induce emesis.
- Administer activated charcoal.

Hospital

- Nasogastric lavage may be useful.
- Super activated charcoal may be given with one dose of cathartic in case of ingestion.
- Provide oxygenation and ventilation as needed.
- Administer hyperbaric oxygen to avoid delayed neurological effects.
- Treat hypotension with IV fluids avoiding fluid overload. Give vasopressors in unresponsive hypotension.
- Correct arterial blood pH with sodium bicarbonate.
- Treat seizures with anticonvulsants and arrhythmias with anti-arrhythmics.
- Use cyanide antidote kit (amyl nitrite, sodium nitrite and sodium thiosulphate) with careful monitoring.
- Hydroxocobalamin (Vitamin B_{12}) is a potential cyanide antidote.

Isopropyl alcohol

It is an aliphatic alcohol used widely in industry and household preparations as a solvent, antiseptic or disinfectant. After-shave lotions, skin lotions, hair tonics and window cleaning fluids may contain isopropyl alcohol. Other names of isopropyl alcohol are isopropanol, propan-1-ol, 2-propanol and secondary propyl alcohol.

Mechanism of toxicity

It causes long lasting CNS depression via formation of its metabolite, acetone. The enzyme alcohol dehydrogenase is involved in its oxidation. Peak plasma level is reached 1hour after ingestion. Its half life is 2.5–3.2 hrs. and 20–50% is excreted unchanged by the kidneys.

Toxic dose

The estimated toxic dose of isopropyl alcohol is 20 ml. Lethal dose in adults is approximately 240 ml. Serum levels of 50 mg/dl are associated with mild toxicity. Ninety ml of 70% can produce blood levels of 100 mg/dl in an adult. Blood levels of 150 mg/dl are associated with coma.

Clinical features

- CNS effects are headache, dizziness, inebriation, ataxia, coma and nystagmus.
- Hypothermia secondary to vasodilation and CNS depression is observed.
- Respiratory failure after large ingestions and aspiration secondary to CNS depression may occur.
- CVS effects include tachycardia/bradycardia and hypotension.
- Metabolic acidosis is mild and the osmolar gap is elevated.
- Hemorrhagic gastritis, vomiting, and hepatocellular damage may be seen.
- Hemolysis, renal failure secondary to severe hypotension and myopathy (with myoglobinuria) is reported.
- Dermal exposure may produce irritation.
- Inhalation may lead to respiratory irritation.

Diagnosis

It is based on history of exposure, presence of mild acidosis and elevated osmolar gap, and characteristic odour of the breath.

Laboratory/Monitoring

- Monitor electrolytes and glucose.
- Obtain serum osmolality, osmolar gap and arterial blood gases.
- Measure acetone levels.
- Monitor liver and renal function tests.

Management

Pre-hospital

- Do not induce emesis.
- Wash the affected area with copious amounts of water, in case of dermal exposure.
- Remove the victim to fresh air if there is an inhalational exposure.

Hospital

- Provide symptomatic and supportive therapy as needed.
- Administer oxygen and provide ventilatory support if required.
- Perform gastric lavage within first 2 hrs. after ingestion with protection of the airway.
- Administer activated charcoal with cathartic.
- Hemodialysis is indicated in severe cases.

Ethylene glycol

It is a colourless, odourless liquid with a pleasant, warm and bitter sweet taste. It is used in industrial solvents, detergents, inks, corrosives, paints, lacquers, pharmaceuticals and in antifreeze preparations.

Mechanism of toxicity

Toxicity is due to its metabolites. It is oxidised by the enzyme alcohol dehydrogenase to glycol aldehyde, followed by rapid conversion to glycolic acid and further to glyoxylic acid. The glyoxylic acid has a short half-life with several metabolic pathways. The major metabolite is formic acid. The glyoxylic acid is converted to glycine and then to carbon dioxide and water in presence of folate. It is also oxidised to oxalic acid and then converted into calcium oxalate resulting in excretion of oxalate crystals in the urine. It conjugates with α-hydroxy-β-ketoadipate in presence of thiamine and magnesium. Ethylene glycol and its metabolites are excreted mainly by the kidneys. The metabolites cause direct renal toxicity and oxalate crystalluria may cause an obstructive uropathy.

Toxic dose

Lethal dose of ethylene glycol is 100 ml.

Clinical features

- After ingestion (30 min.- 4 hrs.), the effects resemble ethanol intoxication with no odour of alcohol in the breath.
- Clinical features include CNS depression associated with cerebral edema and calcium oxalate deposition.
- GI features include nausea, vomiting, abdominal cramps and hematemesis.
- High doses cause confusion, hallucinations, seizures, coma, hypotonia and hyperreflexia, tremors and tetany.
- Ocular findings include decreased pupillary reflexes, nystagmus, decreased visual acuity, optic disc blurring, papilledema, ophthalmoplegia, strabismus, colour blindness and optic atrophy (as observed in methanol intoxication).

- Elevated osmolar gap, high anion gap, lactic acidosis, and hypocalcemia are noted (as in methanol intoxication).
- Cardiopulmonary system involvement occurs 12–48 hrs. after ingestion and the effects include tachypnea, tachycardia, cyanosis, hypertension, and inspiratory rales, cardiac and noncardiogenic pulmonary edema, bronchopneumonia, cardiac dilatation, and arrhythmias.
- Acute renal failure occurs 24–72 hrs. after ingestion. Acute tubular necrosis, renal edema and renal deposition of oxalate crystals contribute to renal failure.

Diagnosis

Diagnosis is based on history of exposure or an unexplained anion gap acidosis. Ethylene glycol poisoning produces hypocalcemia, as well as the appearance of oxalate crystals in the urine.

Laboratory/Monitoring

- Monitor arterial blood gases.
- Measure electrolytes to calculate anion and osmolar gap.
- Perform urinalysis to detect calcium oxalate crystals.
- Monitor blood glucose, BUN, creatinine, CBC and estimate serum calcium levels (severe hypocalcemia may develop).
- Obtain blood ethanol, ethylene glycol and lactic acid levels.
- Monitor ECG.

Management

Pre-hospital

- Induce emesis in alert and awake patients with syrup of ipeac.

Hospital

- Provide symptomatic and supportive therapy.
- Maintain the airway and assist ventilation if required.
- Perform gastric lavage (after controlling seizures and protecting airway).
- Administer sodium bicarbonate in severe and life threatening cases of acidosis and acidemia prior to hemodialysis.
- Ethanol is the specific antidote and is indicated if plasma ethylene glycol levels are >20 mg/dl or in any two of the following conditions, arterial pH < 7.3, serum bicarbonate < 20 mEq/L, osmolar gap >10 mosm/L or urinary oxalate crystals, are present.
- Administer 4-methyl pyrazole, the indications are similar to that of ethanol therapy.
- Perform hemodialysis in case of severe metabolic acidosis, severe electrolyte imbalance, pulmonary edema, renal failure, or when ethylene glycol levels are >50 mg/dl.

Methanol

Methanol (methyl alcohol) is a colourless liquid used in paints, varnish removers, perfumes, household cleaners and as an industrial solvent. Other applications are as an antifreeze, ethanol denaturant, and as a fuel. It is also used in the manufacture of formaldehyde, acetic acid etc.

Mechanism of toxicity

Methanol is biotransformed by the enzyme alcohol dehydrogenase present in the liver and produces formaldehyde. Formaldehyde is converted into formate by enzyme systems aldehyde-dehydrogenase, xanthine oxidase, glyceraldehyde-3-phosphate hydrogenase, catalase, peroxidase, aldehyde oxidase, and glutathione dependent formaldehyde dehydrogenases. Methanol is considered as a cumulative poison due to its slow elimination. Formic acid is thought to be responsible for the ocular toxicity associated with methanol poisoning by inhibiting cytochrome oxidase in the optic nerve and disturbing the flow of axoplasm. The enzyme alcohol dehydrogenase, the principal enzyme involved in the oxidation of ethanol, is also used for oxidation of methanol. Ethanol is preferentially metabolized by the enzyme and hence administration of ethanol delays chemical and biochemical effects of methanol. Ethanol is administered to slow down metabolic transformation of methanol to its toxic products. The elimination half-life of methanol is between 12–20 hrs. in mild cases and 24–30 hrs. in severe intoxications in untreated patients, and this is prolonged to 30-35 hrs. by administration of ethanol. The half-life of methanol can be reduced to 2.5 hrs. by dialysis.

Toxic dose

Methanol itself is harmless, but its metabolites are toxic. 0.25 ml/kg of 100% methanol produces severe toxic effects. 1–2 ml/kg is considered to be lethal. Serum methanol levels of more than 20 mg/dl are toxic and above 40 mg/dl produce severe toxicity.

Clinical features

- Main toxic effect is on nervous system, particularly optic nerves. The condition can progress to permanent blindness.
- Breathlessness, an early sign, is related to unmetabolized methanol.
- In the first few hours inebriation and gastritis are noticed.
- Onset of effects may be delayed for 12–24 hrs.
- Hyperapnea usually develops to compensate for metabolic acidosis.
- Blurred or double vision, constricted visual fields, sharply reduced visual acuity, optic atrophy, blindness, nystagmus, and whiteness in the visual field may be observed.
- Fixed dilated pupils suggest severe poisoning.
- In fatal poisoning marked bradycardia may develop.

- Cardiac failure and severe hypotension may also occur.
- In severe cases tachypnea from metabolic acidosis and in terminal stages sudden respiratory and circulatory failure may occur.
- Seizures, coma and symptoms similar to ethanol intoxication may occur.
- GI effects include abdominal pain, anorexia, nausea and vomiting.
- Hepatic failure is reported in fatal cases.
- Acute renal failure and hematuria are also reported.
- Hypokalemia, hypomagnesemia, and elevated anion gap metabolic acidosis may occur.
- Leukocytosis, coagulation disorders and hyperglycemia are reported following severe methanol intoxication.
- Permanent effects may include basal ganglia infarcts, parkinsonism, toxic encephalopathy and polyneuropathy.

Diagnosis

History of exposure, signs and symptoms, and laboratory findings form the basis of diagnosis. In methanol poisoning increased anion gap is not accounted for by elevated lactate levels.

Laboratory/Monitoring

- Monitor electrolytes, CBC, urinalysis, glucose, BUN, creatinine, serum osmolality and osmolar gap, arterial blood gases, and lactate levels.
- Measure serum pH and anion gap.
- Measure serum ethanol levels on an hourly basis to guide ethanol therapy.
- Estimate serum methanol levels (more than 20 mg/dl are toxic and above 40 mg/dl result in severe intoxication).
- Measure serum formate concentrations (better measure of toxicity).

Management

Pre-hospital

- Induce emesis with syrup of ipecac within an hour of ingestion.
- Lay the patient on a side to prevent aspiration of vomitus.

Hospital

- Provide symptomatic and supportive care as required.
- Ensure clear airway.
- Provide ventilatory support as required.
- Perform gastric lavage if presented within 4 hrs. after ingestion.
- Treat acidosis with sodium bicarbonate with close monitoring of arterial blood gases.

- Ethanol is the specific antidote (orally or as IV infusion). Ethanol therapy is indicated in patients with a history of significant amount of methanol ingestion, metabolic acidosis and an osmolar gap greater than 5–10 mosm/L or if concentration of methanol in blood is greater than 20 mg/dl.
- Hemodialysis is indicated when serum methanol concentration is more than 40 mg/dl, there is significant metabolic acidosis and fluid and electrolyte disturbances despite therapy, visual effects or in case of renal compromise.
- Folic acid may enhance the conversion of formate to carbon dioxide and water.
- 4-methyl pyrazole, an experimental drug, may be tried.

Ethyl alcohol

Ethanol (ethyl alcohol) is a clear and colourless liquid. It is used in alcoholic beverages, toiletries, perfumes, antiseptics, pharmaceuticals and as a solvent. It is one of the most commonly abused substances and a common coingestant with other agents in suicide attempts.

Mechanism of toxicity
The toxic mechanism of ethanol is not specifically known. Some of the manifestations can be related to effects of its metabolite acetaldehyde or to changes in the redox potential of cells. The principal effect of intoxication is on CNS causing depression. It may cause hypoglycemia due to impaired gluconeogenesis in patients with depleted glycogen stores. Liver metabolizes alcohol to acetaldehyde and acetic acid by the enzymes alochol dehydrogenase and aldehyde dehydrogenase.

Toxic dose
Blood levels of 150–300 mg/dl produce toxic effects. Fatal dose is 5-6 g/kg in non-tolerant adults and 3 g/kg in children. Clinical effects in the intolerant ethanol drinker with respect to blood levels are as follows : Blood levels of 30 mg/dl produce mild euphoria and disinhibition. Levels of 50 mg/dl are associated with mild incoordination. Ataxia is observed at blood ethanol levels of 100 mg/dl and drowsiness and confusion at 200 mg/dl. The levels of 300 mg/dl result in stupor, coma while ethanol levels above 400 mg/dl may produce hypoglycemia, hypothermia, respiratory failure, coma and death.

Clinical features

- CNS effects include altered mental status, euphoric feelings, slurred speech, altered perception, impaired judgement, ataxia, incoordination, nystagmus and CNS depression.
- GI effects are nausea, vomiting and abdominal pain.

Diagnosis

History of exposure, characteristic odour of fresh alcohol, odour of acetaldehyde or other metabolites, the clinical effects associated with intoxication and laboratory screens form the basis of diagnosis.

Laboratory/Monitoring

- Measure serum ethanol levels.
- Monitor glucose and electrolytes.
- Obtain chest X-ray, if aspiration is suspected.
- Monitor liver and renal function tests and arterial blood gases.

Management

Pre-hospital

- Lay the patient on side to prevent aspiration of vomitus.
- Induce emesis at the scene if it can be done within a few minutes of exposure.

Hospital

- Provide symptomatic and supportive care.
- Intubate and ventilate if required.
- Perform gastric lavage immediately, in case of a potentially life threatening exposure (within 30 min. of ingestion). Airway protection and seizure control are mandatory prior to gastric decontamination.
- Administer IV fluids as required (avoid excessive use).
- Administer glucose (if bedside glucose level is less than 60 mg/dl) preceded by 100 mg thiamine if chronic alcoholism or malnutrition is suspected.
- Administer naloxone to patients with an abnormal mental status (efficacy is not consistent).

Turpentine oil

Turpentine oil (pine oil) is a volatile, clear, colourless liquid with a characteristic aromatic, penetrating odour. Gum turpentine is a volatile, yellowish, opaque, sticky mass with a characteristic odour. It is an irritant, CNS depressant, with high aspiration hazard. Turpentine is used as a paint thinner, in textile cleaning and in shoe polishes. It is topically used as rubefacient, counter irritant and to treat parasitic infestations.

Toxic dose

An adult dose of 120–180 ml may be fatal if untreated and 15 ml may be fatal in children

Clinical features

- Ingestion produces GI burning, abdominal pain, vomiting, diarrhea, tachycardia, dyspnea, cyanosis and fever.
- Severe ingestions can cause glycosuria, hematuria, albuminuria, anuria, excitement, delirium, ataxia, vertigo, stupor and coma.
- Aspiration hazard is high and may produce chemical pneumonitis and pulmonary edema.
- Death is usually due to respiratory failure.
- Dermal contact may produce contact dermatitis.

Diagnosis

Diagnosis is based on history of exposure and characteristic odour of turpentine oil.

Laboratory/Monitoring

- Consider chest X-ray in symptomatic patients.
- Monitor CBC and renal function tests.

Management

Pre-hospital

- Do not induce emesis.

Hospital

- Do not perform gastric lavage if ingestion is < 2 ml/kg.
- Treatment includes support of cardiovascular or respiratory functions as needed.
- Observe for pneumonitis.
- All asymptomatic patients should be observed for 6 hrs. before discharging.

Agents producing methemoglobinemia

Methemoglobin is an oxidised form of hemoglobin. This abnormal hemoglobin is incapable of carrying oxygen to the cells. Both congenital and acquired methemoglobinemia are observed. Exposure to a wide variety of drugs and chemicals can induce methemoglobinemia. Toxic exposures from acetanilid, air freshners, aminosalicylic acid, aniline, benzocaine, bismuth, chlorates, chloroquine, chromates, copper, dapsone, inks, lidocaine, menthol, methylene blue, naphthalene, nitrates, nitrites, nitrobenzene, nitroprusside, phenacetin, phenobarbital, phenols, phenytoin, piperazine, potassium permanganate, procaine, quinolones, resorcinol, shoe polish, silver nitrate, sodium nitrate, sulphonamides, thiocyanates, trimethoprim, vitamin K, trinitrotoluene, varnishes, water from contaminated wells etc. may induce methemoglobinemia.

Mechanism of toxicity

An oxidant substance oxidises ferrous iron (Fe^{2+}) in the hemoglobin to ferric (Fe^{3+}) methemoglobin, which is incapable of carrying oxygen. In addition to the impaired oxygen carrying capacity of blood, methemoglobin enhances the affinity of hemoglobin for oxygen, thereby reducing the oxygen delivery to the tissues. Generally, in normal individuals, the methemoglobin level is maintained below 1% by an NADH dependent methemoglobin reductase enzyme. Another enzyme, NADPH reductase is effective in reducing ferric iron in methemoglobin to ferrous form in presence of an electron donating cofactor, methylene blue. This is the basis of using methylene blue in methemoglobinemia. This system rapidly converts methemoglobin to hemoglobin.

Toxic dose

Estimates of toxic/lethal amounts of any particular drug or chemical is of little value due to wide variation in individual susceptibility to methemoglobin formation. However, methemoglobin (Meth. Hb) levels can be well correlated with toxic effects. Meth. Hb levels below 15% are usually asymptomatic. Levels of 15–20% are associated with cyanosis and mild symptoms. Marked cyanosis and moderate symptoms are noticed with Meth. Hb levels of 20–45% and severe cyanosis and severe toxic effects are observed when the levels are 45–70%. Meth Hb levels above 70% are considered to be lethal.

Clinical features

- Central cyanosis is unresponsive to supplemental oxygen therapy.
- Headache, lethargy, dizziness, fatigue, syncope, dyspnea, CNS depression, seizures, arrhythmias and shock may be caused.

Meth. Hb levels of:
- 15–20% generally produce cyanosis and chocolate-brown blood.
- 20–45% are associated with headache, lethargy, dizziness, fatigue, syncope, dyspnea.
- 45–55% lead to increased CNS depression and metabolic acidosis.
- 55–70% result in coma, seizures, arrhythmias and shock.
- Above 70% show high incidence of mortality even after treatment.

Diagnosis

Cyanosis unresponsive to oxygen therapy and chocolate brown colour of blood are indicative of methemoglobinemia. Put a drop of blood on a filter paper and compare with normal blood.

Laboratory/Monitoring

- Measure methemoglobin levels.
- Monitor electrolytes, arterial blood gases and hemoglobin.
- Obtain chest X-ray and monitor ECG.

Management

Pre-hospital

- Move the patient to fresh air.
- Transport to a health care facility immediately.

Hospital

- Provide supportive care as required.
- Administer humidified supplemental oxygen. Assist ventilation as required.
- Methylene blue is the specific antidote. Administer in patients with Meth. Hb levels more than 30% and in symptomatic patients (other than cyanosis).
- Administer hyperbaric oxygen in very serious cases that do not respond rapidly to antidotal therapy. It is contraindicated in hemodynamically unstable patients. Adverse effects include oxygen toxicity, barotrauma, pneumothorax and seizures and all are treated by withdrawing hyperbaric therapy.
- Perform exchange transfusion in severe cases where methylene blue is contraindicated.
- Treat hypotension with hypotonic fluids and vasopressors if required.

Agents producing sulfhemoglobinemia

Sulfhemoglobin (SHb) is an abnormal hemoglobin. It is generally self limiting following cessation of the implicated agent, and resolves with the turnover of new red blood cells. It decreases oxyhemoglobin saturation and is unresponsive to methylene blue, and hence patients may continue to appear cyanotic even after receiving the antidote. Various drugs and chemicals can induce sulfhemoglobinemia. Sulfhemoglobinemia is induced by the ingestion of phenacetin, acetanilid, sulfonamides, metoclopramide and dapsone. Hydrogen sulphide and combustion products of sulphur compounds also induce sulfhemoglobinemia.

Mechanism of toxicity

SHb is a hemoglobin molecule altered by the addition of a sulphur atom in the porphyrin ring rendering it incapable of carrying oxygen. SHb, unlike methemoglobin, is not converted to normal hemoglobin and persists until the red blood cells are broken down by the reticuloendothelial system. Since the life of RBC is about 120 days, the prognosis may be delayed without treatment.

Toxic dose

Sulfhemoglobin levels of 2–3% may produce noticeable cyanosis.

Clinical features

- Clinical cyanosis with no respiratory or cardiovascular involvement is observed.
- Severe dyspnea is rare, unless accompanied by methemoglobinemia. SHb levels of:
- 5–15% cause cyanosis without any additional symptoms.
- Above 15% produce nonspecific symptoms like nausea, headache, and palpitations.
- 50–60% worsen the cardiopulmonary symptoms and possible obtundation.
- 70–80% are fatal.

Laboratory/Monitoring

- Monitor arterial blood gases and electrolytes.
- Estimate sulfhemoglobin levels.
- Obtain chest X-ray and monitor ECG.

Management

Pre-hospital

- Move the patient to fresh air.

Hospital

- Provide symptomatic and supportive care.
- Administer humidified supplemental oxygen to all cyanotic patients.
- Give hyperbaric oxygen in severe cases. It is contraindicated in hemodynamically unstable patients. Adverse effects include oxygen toxicity, barotrauma, pneumothorax and seizures and all are treated by withdrawing hyperbaric therapy.
- In severe poisonings consider exchange transfusion.
- Methylene blue has no role in the treatment of sulfhemoglobinemia.

8. Environmental Toxins

Cannabis

Marijuana is the common name for *Cannabis sativa*. It contains a number of cannabinoids. Δ^9-tetrahydrocannabinol (THC) is the main psychoactive agent. The narcotic drugs Bhang, Hashish, Ganja and Charas are the dried flowering and fruiting tops of the pistillate plants of *Cannabis sativa* from which no resin has been removed. Bhang, Ganja and Charas were habitually used by millions of people in India, but in recent years, due to statutory restrictions, their use is progressively being restricted. Dried leaves and flowering shoots are the parts mainly used. Hashish, Bhang and Hashish oil are the other cannabis products containing more concentrated forms of the plant alkaloids. They are used as astringent, tonic, aphrodisiac, intoxicant, analgesic, abortifacient etc. They are also used in convulsions, otalgia, and somatalgia. The bark of the plant is useful in inflammations, haemorrhoids and hydrocele, however, it is toxic. The seeds are carminative, astringent, aphrodisiac, antiemetic and antiinflammatory. Bhang, Siddhi, Sabji or Patti are the other names of this product.

Toxic dose
The acute oral toxicity of cannabis as an intoxicant is low. Estimated lethal dose of cannabis in humans is 30 mg/kg of absorbed cannabis, otherwise the lethal dose is not known. Marijuana or Grass contains 1-5% THC. Hashish or Charas contains 10% and hashish oil contains 50% or more of THC.

Clinical features
- Cannabis affects the brain and the adverse effects associated with the use of cannabis are altered sensorium, blood pressure changes, blurred vision, decreased coordination, dizziness, dry mouth and eyes, hallucinations, heart rate changes, respiratory allergy, sedation, skin rash, somnolence etc.
- Higher doses produce coma and death from cardiac failure.
- Excessive use causes dyspepsia, cough, impotence, melencholy, dropsy, hyperpyrexia and insanity.
- Injection results in severe headache, dizziness, irregular breathing, hyperthermia, hypotension, tachycardia and unconsciousness.

- Nausea, vomiting, diarrhea, and abdominal pain may occur.
- Muscle pain, albuminuria, and renal failure are the other features.
- In case of inhalation the onset of effects is seen within 10 minutes.
- Toxic effects start within 30-60 min. after ingestion.

Diagnosis
It is based on history of exposure and characteristic features.

Laboratory/Monitoring

- Monitor ECG.
- Estimate blood glucose levels.

Management

Pre-hospital

- Induce emesis with syrup of ipecac, if it can be given immediately (within minutes) after ingestion.
- Give activated charcoal.
- Lay unconscious or drowsy patient on one side.
- Keep anxious and confused patient in a quiet room.
- Shift the patient immediately to a health care facility if cannabis has been injected.

Hospital

- Provide supportive care as in case of a sedative-hypnotic poisoning.
- Support respiration, blood pressure and other functions as needed.
- Give benzodiazepines to treat agitation, panic or disorientation.
- Administer haloperidol to treat psychotic features.
- Administer propranolol only to very severe cases of sinus tachycardia. Usually treatment is not required.

Datura

This plant commonly called "Thorn apple" shows anticholinergic properties. Though all parts are toxic but the seeds are most noxious. The seeds are used as narcotic, anodyne, antispasmodic, intoxicant and emetic, and also to treat asthma, cough, fever, ulcers and skin diseases. The roots are used to cure insanity and to treat bites from rabid dogs. A poultice made from the leaves is used for ophthalmodynia, otalgia, lumbago, sciatica, neuralgia, mumps and painful swellings. The juice of the leaves is used for epilepsy and dandruff. The seeds are aphrodisiac and narcotic and are useful in odontalgia and otalgia.

Mechanism of toxicity

The alkaloids present in the plant are atropine and hyoscine, both of which have anticholinergic effects. They antagonize the effects of acetylcholine at peripheral, muscarinic and central receptors. Exocrine glands such as those responsible for sweating and salivation as well as smooth and cardiac muscles are affected.

Toxic dose

Ingestion of a single seed is toxic. Ingestion of 100 seeds may be fatal. Ingestion of 4 g of the plant material may be lethal to a child.

Clinical features

- Anticholinergic toxidrome is produced with intoxication.
- Peripheral symptoms include tachycardia, dry flushed skin and mucous membranes, mydriasis, hyperpyrexia, urinary retention, decreased bowel sounds, hypotension/hypertension, arrhythmias, delirium, disorientation, frank psychosis and ataxia.
- Stupor, convulsions and coma are observed in very severe cases.
- Ingestion of seeds results in immediate vomiting, bitter taste, dry mouth, burning pain in epigastrium and dysphagia.
- Decreased gastrointestinal motility with loss of bowel sounds, urinary retention, anxiety, disorientation, hyperactivity, delirium, hallucinations, mental status depression, seizures and coma may be observed.
- Severe toxicity may result in respiratory failure and cardiovascular collapse.
- Mild to moderate toxicity usually resolves within 1-2 days. (Rarely lasts as long as 2 weeks).

Diagnosis

The diagnosis is based on history of exposure and presence of characteristic features like dilated pupils and dry flushed skin.

Laboratory/Monitoring

- Monitor electrolytes, glucose and arterial blood gases.
- Monitor ECG.

Management

Pre-hospital

- Emesis is useful if induced within 30 min. of ingestion.
- Administer activated charcoal.

Hospital

- Maintain the airway and assist ventilation if required.
- Gastric decontamination may be useful even in patients presenting 12-24 hrs. following ingestion, due to the decreased GI motility.
- Treat hyperthermia, seizures and coma conservatively.
- Administer 'physostigmine' in severe poisonings (severe delirium, seizures, tachycardia or arrhythmias unresponsive to standard antiarrhythmics).
- Propranolol may be useful for significant arrhythmias.
- Control hyperthermia using external cooling.

Argemone

Argemone mexicana (Prickly poppy) grows all over the country as a wild plant. On extraction, the seeds yield a pale-yellow liquid which may be used for lamps. This is known as argemone oil or katakar oil. Argemone oil is frequently used as an adulterant in cooking oils especially mustard oil. Argemone seeds as such are not taken orally. Dihydrosanguinarine (87%) and sanguinarine (5%) of the total alkaloids are the major alkaloids present in the argemone oil. Ingestion of cooking oils contaminated with 'argemone oil' produces "epidemic dropsy".

Toxic dose

0.01% of argemone seed oil in an edible oil if consumed for 5-20 days produces subacute poisoning.

Clinical features

- Epidemic dropsy is characterized by onset of pedal edema, tenderness, erythema and rash over the edematous parts.
- GI effects include diarrhea, vomiting, abdominal pain and tenesmus.
- Cardiovascular effects include palpitations, tachycardia, wide pulse pressure, congestive heart failure, and even death in severe cases.
- Low grade fever may be present.
- Hepatomegaly may occur.
- Ocular effects include glaucoma and retinal vascular changes (dilated, tortuous vessels and superficial retinal hemorrhage).
- Bronchitis and hair loss are also reported.

Diagnosis

Diagnosis is based on history of exposure and characteristic features of poisoning. More than one member of the family is generally affected from the consumption of the adulterated oil and poisonings reach epidemic proportions.

Laboratory/Monitoring

- Monitor ECG and chest X-ray.
- Detect and estimate argemone oil (alkaloids) in suspected oil.
- Estimation of alkaloids in blood and urine may be useful.

Management

- There is no established treatment protocol.
- Discontinue use of adulterated oil, if any, with immediate effect.
- The mainstay of therapy is symptomatic and supportive care.
- Trials of diuretics and steroids have been attempted.
- There is no specific antidote and decontamination is generally not required.
- Administration of antioxidants flavin, β-carotene and α-tocopherol may be useful for reducing the argemone oil induced hepatotoxicity.

Oleander

Thevetia neriifolia (yellow oleander) is an ornamental shrub widespread in the tropical and subtropical regions. Poisoning can occur after accidental ingestion, suicide, homicide or inhalation of smoke from burning of oleander. Various parts of the plant have been used in folk medicine, as insecticides and fish poisons. All parts of the plant contain cardiac glycosides. Seeds have highest concentration of the toxins.

Mechanism of toxicity

It produces high grade heart block with significant interference of ATPase mediated sodium potassium pump mechanism. Electrical conduction is interfered with decrease in intracellular potassium resulting in progressive electrical changes. Complete loss of normal myocardial electrical function occurs with asystole. Hyperkalemia and loss of excitability of cardiac tissue results from massive overdose.

Toxic dose

There is a marked variability in effects from the ingestion of *T. neriifolia* (cardiac glycosides). Toxic dose in adults is 2 seeds and fatality may be produced by the ingestion of 8-10 seeds.

Clinical features

- Effects of the glycosides are similar to that of digitalis but with a more rapid onset.
- Ingestion causes burning sensation in mouth, tingling of tongue, dryness of throat, nausea, vomiting and diarrhea, giddiness or dizziness.
- Common cardiac features are ECG changes, AV block and bradycardia. ST depression, ectopic beats and palpitations are also seen.

- Blood pressure may initially be elevated but would fall later due to bradycardia.
- Arrhythmias and hyperkalemia may be uncontrollable leading to fatality.

Laboratory/Monitoring

- Monitor serum potassium, blood urea, and arterial blood gases.
- Monitor serum calcium and magnesium in symptomatic patients.
- Obtain a base line ECG even in asymptomatic patients.

Management

Pre-hospital

- Induce emesis with syrup of ipecac.
- Transport immediately to a health care facility.

Hospital

- The treatment is symptomatic and supportive.
- Give cholestyramine to reduce absorption of cardiac glycosides from the gut.
- Give IV fluids.
- A pacemaker may be used if third degree heart block occurs. It is not required in case of a first degree block without ventricular extra systoles and a non-deteriorating condition.
- Low dose phenytoin improves atrio-ventricular conduction and may terminate heart block and increase heart rate.
- Treat hyperkalemia.
- Metabolic acidosis with sodium bicarbonate.
- Administer atropine to maintain cardiac output. It is used for restoring atrial activity and increasing heart rate.
- Give lignocaine to treat ventricular arrhythmias.
- There is no specific antidote.

Snake bites

There are about 200 species of snakes in India, of which 52 are poisonous. The commonly encountered snake bite envenomations in India are of elapids (Cobra and Krait) or viperides (Saw scaled viper and Russel's viper). The degree of envenomation is influenced by size and species of the snake, age and size of the victim and also the bite may be severe after hybernation. Bites on upper extremity are more serious than lower. Hemophilia, concurrent anticoagulant therapy or peptic ulceration predispose a victim to hemorrhage. Menstrual bleeding may be enhanced and pregnant woman may abort.

Toxic dose

A single bite can be lethal. However, most of the bites do not result in envenomation.

Mechanism of toxicity

Elapidae (Cobra and Krait)
Venom produces neurotoxic effects and sometimes cardiovascular effects are also noticed. Onset of effects can be within minutes but these usually develop after a few hours of being bitten.

Viperidae (Saw scaled viper and Russel's viper)
Cytotoxic and hemotoxic effects are common. Hemorrhages are aggravated by proteolysis, thrombocytopenia and other coagulation disturbances. Endothelial cell lining of blood vessels is destroyed by haemorrhagins leading to extravasation.

Clinical features

Elapidae

- Tachycardia and mild hypertension are initially common due to anxiety or toxic effect.
- Swelling at the site of bite does not usually appear for 2-3 hrs. after the bite. There is not much pain or swelling at the site of bite.
- Sleepiness is followed by ptosis and impaired vision (ophthalmoplegia).
- Slurred speech, difficulty in swallowing and hypersalivation may be observed. In severe cases aspiration of oral secretions can occur.
- Paresthesias, generalized muscle weakness, respiratory impairment and arrest and pulmonary edema may be produced.

Viperidae

- Severe pain is noticed within minutes, followed by swelling at the site of bite (within 15-30 min.).
- At times, there is a blood stained discharge from the wound. These effects resolve within 30-60 min.
- Swelling and oozing starts within 24-36 hrs. and the victim starts bleeding from the gums, nose, kidneys and other sites.
- In severe cases acute renal failure may occur.
- Early shock is probably due to vasodilation while late shock may be precipitated by massive GI hemorrhage or due to acute pituitary failure.

Diagnosis
Diagnosis should be based on the identification of the snake, local examination of fang marks and signs and symptoms associated with envenomation, if any.

In case of Elapid bite envenomations local effects are moderate, venom is neurotoxic (cardiotoxicity and vasculotoxicity are rare), onset of effects is within 1-12 hours and two puncture marks at the site of bite may be observed on careful examination with a hand lens.

Viperids have hollow, short, erectile, fixed and grooved fangs and produce typical fang mark as a puncture or scratch. Local effects are severe. Vasculotoxicity and coagulopathy are common, neurotoxicity is rare. Onset of effects is within 1-24 hours.

Laboratory/Monitoring

- Blood investigations include grouping, cross matching, clotting-time, clot reaction time, total leukocyte counts, platelet counts, prothrombin time.
- Monitor arterial blood gases, renal and liver function tests and electrolytes.
- Perform urinalysis and monitor urine output and myoglobinuria.
- Measurement of fibrin degradation products may give an early clue to intravascular coagulation.
- Monitor cardiac status continuously.

Management

Pre-hospital

- Reassure the patient and apply ligature a few centimeters above the site of bite, tightened to the extent that a finger can pass through underneath it.
- Clean the wound with soap and water.
- Immobilize the bitten limb.

Hospital

- Maintain the airway and assist ventilation as required.
- Remove ligature slowly.
- Administer IV fluids.
- Antisnake venom (ASV) is the antidote.
- Perform sensitivity test before using ASV.
- Monitor the patient for evidence of allergic reactions throughout infusion of ASV.
- Continue administration of antivenin in selected cases of severe envenomations even in presence of allergic reactions with concomitant use of corticosteroids, epinephrine and antihistamines. Slowing the rate of infusion of the antivenin or further dilution can reduce severity of allergic reactions.
- Children need as much or more ASV as adults, but the total volume of diluent is reduced.
- Dose of ASV depends on clinical effects rather than age or weight.
- In Cobra bite envenomations administer neostigmine at intervals of half an hour preceded by atropine to reverse muscular paralysis.

9. Scorpion, Wasp and Bee Stings

Scorpion sting

Scorpions are the members of order scorpionida which has many families, genera and species. They are the most primitive and oldest members of the terrestrial arachnids. Usually they are nocturnal predators, seeking moist and cool areas and inhabiting the subtropical and tropical parts of the globe and are more active in summer and rainy season. Scorpions differ in colour from straw yellow or light brown to black.

All scorpions have a pair of venom glands in bulbous terminal segment of the tail called 'telson' located anterior to the stinger. The glands produce venom which is injected with the sting. The virulence of the venom varies in different species. Due to the difference in susceptibility and the virulence of the species, the reactions to sting vary in severity from painful prick to death in children. A stinger may cause single puncture wound or a series if struck several times in quick succession. Fingers, hands, toes and legs are commonly stung. There are a number of venomous scropions and some of the most common ones include species of *Buthus* (India) and *Centurus* (USA). The common poisonous scorpions found in India are *Mesobuthus tamulus* (common Indian red scorpion) and *Palamnieus swammerdami* and *P. gravimamus* (black scorpion). *Heterometris bengalensis* is a native of Eastern India found especially around West Bengal. Scorpion stings are common in rural India mainly in the Southern states.

Mechanism of toxicity

The composition and toxicity of scorpion venom varies widely. Generally, the venom consists of ten or more basic neurotoxic proteins and atleast six non proteins. Most of the toxins affect the sodium channels of the excitable cells by retarding inactivation or enhancing activation. A few of these toxins affect the potassium channels also. Severe autonomic and central nervous system manifestations occur because the venom is a potent sodium channel activator. There is a massive release of catecholamines from the nerve endings and adrenal glands into the circulation, besides the direct effect on heart. Severe cardiac, respiratory and pancreatic dysfunction may occur resulting in multisystem organ failure and death.

Clinical features

- Mild to severe pain results at the site of the sting with or without the development of systemic features.
- Symptoms occuring within 2-12 hrs. of sting include hypertension, nausea, vomiting, excessive salivation, diaphoresis, headache, agitation or paresthesias, restlessness, mydriasis, priapism, respiratory distress and insufficiency. Pulmonary edema may be delayed in onset upto 24-72 hrs.
- Tachycardia and hypertension are the common early signs.
- Bradycardia, hypotension, arrhythmias, left ventricular dysfunction, cardiomyopathy and ECG changes are less common.
- Some unusual manifestations include pancreatitis, hemolysis, acute renal failure, rhabdomyolysis, disseminated intravascular coagulation and seizures.
- Recovery usually occurs within 12-36 hrs. in nonfatal cases.

Diagnosis

The patient should have seen the scorpion. The patients almost always show a positive "tap test" when tapping on the sting site usually produces severe pain.

Laboratory/Monitoring

- No laboratory studies need to be done for mild envenomations.
- For severe envenomations monitor CBC, electrolytes, glucose, BUN, creatinine, coagulation profile and arterial blood gases.
- Monitor blood pressure, heart rate, ECG and respiratory status continuously.

Management

Pre-hospital

- Do not apply tourniquets or perform local incisions or suction.
- Put ice over the wound intermittently. Do not immerse the extremity in ice.
- Immobilize the patient and withhold food during first 8-12 hrs.

Hospital

- Treatment is supportive and symptomatic.
- Maintain the airway and assist ventilation if necessary, administer supplemental oxygen.
- Give IV fluids to correct fluid loss.
- Treat hypertension with prazosin and nifedipine.

- Role of corticosteroids in pulmonary edema is controversial.
- Role of antivenins is controversial.

Wasp and Bee stings

The order hymenoptera consists of a large group of insects that include ants, honey bees, bumble bees, wasps, yellow jackets and hornets. Most bees sting only when disturbed or when the hive is threatened. The venom sac is attached to the stinger and squeezing or exerting pressure on the venom sac may force venom into the wound. The honey bee stings only once, as the stinger is barbed and catches in the victim's skin, resulting in tearing of the stinger and venom sac from the bee's body as it pulls away. The insect dies as it flies away. The bumble, bees, wasps, hornets and yellow jackets have unbarbed stinger that remains functionally intact after a sting, thus capable of multiple stings.

Mechanism of toxicity

The venoms of the hymenoptera are mixtures of several antigens, non-immunologic small peptides and vasoactive amines. The known protein and peptide components in honey bee and vespid venom include phospholipase A_2, hyaluronidase, acid phosphatase, mellitin, apamin, MCD peptide (honey bee); phospholipase-A, B, hyaluronidase, antigen-5, kinin and mastoparan (wasps). Mellitin present in relatively high concentrations in bee venom is responsible for much of the local pain caused by the sting and alters membrane integrity. Phospholipase A_2 induces red cell hemolysis after mellitin has disrupted the cell membrane. Mast cell degranulating peptide results in mast cell release of histamine and hyaluronidase in addition to acting as an allergen, causes disruption of hyaluronic acid connective tissue matrix allowing for spread of venom into tissue. Peptide neurotoxin, apamin has a profound effect on spinal cord function, causing hyperactivity, muscle spasms and seizures. The non-allergenic amines which are released include acetylcholine, histamine, catecholamines (bee venom); histamine, catecholamines and serotonin (wasps). They have inflammatory and vasoactive properties that contribute to normal focal reaction to a sting and may hasten absorption of venom allergens.

Toxic dose

The range of toxicity from a non-immunological reaction is venom dose-dependent extending from trivial to death in case of massive attacks. The toxic response is highly variable depending on individual sensitivity. Wasps have the ability to sting several times thereby increasing the venom load. Twenty or more stings from a wasp may cause severe morbidity or death. Although more than 1000 honey bee stings have been incurred with survival, 150 or more stings have caused severe morbidity and death. Several thousand stings can result from massive attacks by bees while massive wasp attacks range from ten to hundreds of stings. A honey bee can inject 50-100 μg of venom through one sting.

Clinical features

- Non allergic local reaction includes localized severe pain, wheal formation, irritation, itching, redness at the site of sting, vesiculation and blisters.
- Stings in mouth or throat leading to local edema may cause respiratory obstruction.
- Multiple stings or very rarely single sting may produce vomiting, diarrhea, edema, fatigue, headache, hypotension, seizures, unconsciousness, syncope, dyspnea, rhabdomyolysis, coagalopathy and death.
- Hypersensivity (anaphylactic) reactions cause extensive local swelling and urticaria.
- Even one sting may cause a serious reaction in a hypersensitive individual.
- Systemic allergic reactions which may occur within 30 min. of a sting include generalized urticaria, erythema, pruritus, angioedema, edema of tongue, epiglottis, and larynx, bronchial constriction causing dyspnea, stridor, dysphagia or wheezing and or cardiovascular collapse, hypotension and loss of consciousness.
- Cause of death is usually respiratory obstruction, cardiovascular collapse or both.
- Delayed toxic reactions are rare. Such patients are asymptomatic after a massive bee envenomation with normal initial laboratory results but later develop hemolysis, coagulopathy, thrombocytopenia, rhabdomyolysis, liver dysfunction and disseminated intravascular coagulation.
- Corneal stings may cause corneal edema, ulceration, hyperemia, pain, scarring and linear keratitis.
- External eye stings cause localized pain, swelling, tearing, hyperemia and conjunctival chemosis.
- Multiple bee stings cause hypertension and tachycardia.

Diagnosis

Diagnosis is based on the history of exposure and typical findings.

Laboratory/Monitoring

- Monitor cardiac status continuously.

Management

Pre-hospital

- Remove the retained stinger and venom sac carefully as soon as possible by gentle scraping with a piece of cardboard, knife, blade or other blunt edged device.
- Do not squeeze the stinger with forceps or fingers as more venom will be released.
- Wash the sting area with soap and water.
- In case an extremity is involved, apply a loose constriction band proximal to the sting site.
- Apply ice packs locally at the sting site which may decrease the intensity of swelling.

Hospital

- Painful localized tissue response resolves without therapy in a few hours.
- Treat mild cases with antihistamines with or without epinephrine.
- For symptomatic relief of pain apply ice, papain or creams containing antihistamines or corticosteroids.
- In severe cases manage airway and assist ventilation, give supplemental oxygen. Give IV epinephrine (1:10,000 or 1:100,000 soln.) depending upon patient's BP.
- Give IV fluids and vasopressors in face of shock.
- Treat mild to severe bronchospam with bronchodilators.
- Corticosteroids can be given.
- Life threatening manifestations of anaphylaxis may recur in 20% of patients following an asymptomatic interval of 8-12 hrs. after treatment of the initial episode.
- Observe patients for at least 12 hrs. after the onset of the initial anaphylactic episode.
- Manage large local allergic reactions with a brief tapering course of a corticosteroid.
- Serum sickness-like response with symptoms of fever, arthralgia, urticaria, angioedema may occur 1-2 weeks after a sting.

10. Mushrooms and Food Poisoning

Mushrooms

Mushroom or Toad stool is a common name for the fruit of certain kinds of fungi. Of the possible 10,000 species of mushrooms occuring worldwide, only about 50 to 100 are known to be toxic. Mushrooms can be categorised into several groups based on the toxins they contain and the signs and symptoms of toxicity. Seven groups of toxins have been identified i.e. cyclopeptide, monomethylhydrazine, muscarine, coprine, ibotonic acid, psilocybin and gastrointestinal toxin in various kinds of mushrooms.

Cyclopeptide containing mushrooms are responsible for over 90% of all deaths due to mushrooms. There are three groups of cyclopeptides namely phallotoxins, amatoxins and virotoxins. All these cyclopeptides are heat-stable and insoluble in water. Amatoxins are the most toxic in humans. They are actively absorbed and are potent hepatotoxins. Phallotoxins and virtoxins are probably not absorbed from the gastrointestinal tract and hence are less toxic.

Monomethylhydrazine containing mushrooms are found in spring and easily recognised by their brain like appearance. They contain monomethyl hydrazine group which inhibits GABA in the CNS.

Muscarine containing mushrooms include *Amanita* (Death Cap) and *Clitocybe* species. Mushrooms known as "Inky caps" contain coprine which is an amino acid with disulfiram like effect. They block acetaldehyde dehydrogenase causing accumulation of acetaldehyde and accompanying adverse effects when consumed with alcohol. Ibotonic acid and muscimol containing mushrooms include some *Amanita* species which contain both the toxins. They produce hallucinations and anticholinergic effects. Psilocybin containing mushrooms are chemically similar to serotonin. Psilocybin and psilocin are similar to LSD and produce CNS effects.

Mechanism of toxicity

There are various mechanisms of toxicity depending on the toxin present in a particular species. However, the majority of toxic incidents are caused by gastrointestinal irritants that produce vomiting and diarrhea.

Toxic dose

One death cap (Am*anita phalloides*) can cause death. 0.1 mg/kg of amatoxin is considered lethal. At least 15 to 20 galerina mushrooms are needed to cause death. Ingestion of just a few gastrointestinal irritant mushrooms can produce marked gastroenteritis.

Clinical features

Symptoms noted 3 hrs. post ingestion

Coprine Group

- Ingestion produces flushing of the face and trunk, palpitations, dyspnea, chest pain, diaphoresis and hypotension (secondary to vasodilation).
- The reaction may occur or may be precipitated after the ingestion of ethanol as long as 1 week after consumption of C*oprinus atramentarius*.

Muscarine Group

- Cholinergic syndrome comprising of vomiting, miosis, salivation, lacrimation, bronchorrhoea, bronchospasm, bradycardia, diarrhea and urinary retention may be observed.
- Seizures may occur in severe cases.

Ibotonic acid and Muscimol Group

- Ingestion produces alcohol like intoxication, ataxia, spontaneous jerking movements and delirium.
- Seizures and coma may develop in severe cases.

Psilocybin Group

- In addition to a psychedelic experience, tachycardia, mydriasis and paresthesias commonly develop and seizures occur rarely.
- The initial episode lasts for 4 to 6 hrs.
- In children, fever (102–106°F) may develop with intermittent tonic-clonic seizures.

Gastrointestinal Irritant Group

- Onset of symptoms is usually within 30 min. to 3 hrs. of ingestion and includes nausea, vomiting, diarrhea, malaise and severe epigastric pain.
- Inter and intra individual variation occurs. The same species may cause symptoms in one person at one time and not at another time (intra individual variation).

Symptoms noted more than 6 hrs. after ingestion

Cyclopeptide group

- *Amanita* poisoning develops in four stages.
- The first phase is a latent period of 6 to 12 hrs. and is of diagnostic value. In mixed mushroom ingestion, symptoms may develop within 3 hrs.
- The second or gastrointestinal phase begins in 6 to 12 hrs. and is characterized by nausea, vomiting, abdominal pain and cholera like diarrhea with concurrent dehydration and hypoglycemia.
- The third phase is another period of latency. Although the patient feels better when the gastrointestinal phase is over, liver injury becomes evident at this stage by the rise in ALT, AST, LDH and abnormal coagulation profile. A rapid fall of coagulation factors usually indicates poor prognosis.
- The fourth or hepatic phase follows. During this period, fulminant hepatic failure and possibly acute renal failure become clinically apparent.
- The patient may progress to hepatic encephalopathy, coma and death

Monomethylhydrazine group

- Symptoms are usually mild and include vomiting, diarrhea, dizziness, fatigue and muscle cramps.
- Delirium, coma and seizures may develop in severe cases.
- Methemoglobinemia and hemolysis may be life threatening.
- Pancreatitis may develop.

Symptoms noted at more than 24 hrs. after ingestion

The orelline/orellanine group produces late-onset nausea, vomiting, oliguria and renal failure.

Diagnosis

Diagnosis is based on history of ingestion combined with clinical presentation and identification of the mushroom (if possible).

Laboratory/Monitoring

- Monitor hepatic and renal functions for at least 48 hrs.
- Monitor electrolytes, glucose and prothrombin time.
- Specific toxin levels are not available.

Management

Pre-hospital

- Do not induce emesis in patients who have already developed spontaneous vomiting.
- Emesis is most effective if initiated within 30 min. of ingestion.

Hospital

- Provide supportive and symptomatic care.
- Administer activated charcoal and a cathartic.
- Gastric emptying is not necessary if activated charcoal can be given promptly.
- Poisoning due to cyclopeptide containing mushrooms does not require gastric lavage and cathartic.
- Treat hypotension with IV fluids.
- Give antiemetics as required.
- Penicillin and silibinin are considered to protect against action of the toxins on liver for cyclopeptide containing mushrooms.
- Control seizures with anticonvulsants.
- Role of steroids is suggested.
- Administration of pyridoxine may help in limiting the toxicity, particularly seizures in poisoning by monomethylhydrazine containing mushrooms.
- Atropine may alleviate cholinergic symptoms in muscarine containing mushroom intoxication.
- Definite signs of anticholinergic symptoms due to ibotonic acid or muscimol containing mushrooms may improve with physostigmine.
- Thiotic acid for mushrooms of cyclopeptide group is no longer recommended.
- Administer penicillin by continuous IV infusion.
- Give methylene blue if methemoglobin levels are greater than 30%.
- There is no specific antidote for mushroom poisoning.

Food poisoning

Bacterial pathogens are the commonest etiologic agents for food poisoning. Bacterial food poisoning manifested by acute gastroenteritis is a disturbance of the gastrointestinal tract with abdominal pain and diarrhea. Gastroenteritis is caused by ingestion of contaminated vegetables, fruits, salad, fried rice, corn flour, milk, cheese, meat, egg products or water. In general, bacterial food poisoning is relatively mild and self-limiting with recovery within a period of 24 hrs. However, severe and even fatal poisoning may occur with *Salmonellosis or Botulism.* Food poisoning may also be caused by a direct infection or invasion of the intestines by *E.coli* or *Salmonella* species. Other causes of food poisoning by direct bacterial infection include *Shigella* (bacillary dysentery), *Streptococcus faecali* and *Yersinia enterocolitica.* Food poisoning may also be caused by viruses (eg rotavirus in children) and protozoa, such as *Entamoeba histolytica* (amoebiasis) and *Giardia lamblia* (giardiasis). Toxic contaminants like PCBs, heavy metals or natural toxic substance (akee fruit) etc. may also cause food poisoning. The most commonly reported pathogens include **Staphylococcus species, Clostridium perfringens, Bacillus cereus, and Campylobacter jejuni.**

Mechanism of toxicity

Gastroenteritis may be caused by invasive bacterial infection of the intestinal mucosa or by a toxin elaborated by bacteria. Bacterial toxins may be preformed in food that is improperly prepared and stored before use or may be produced in the gut by the bacteria after they are ingested.

Toxic dose

The toxic dose depends on the type of bacteria or toxin and its concentration in the ingested food as well as individual susceptibility or resistance. Some of the preferred toxins (eg S*taphylococcal* toxin) are heat resistant and once in the food, are not removed by cooking or boiling.

Clinical features

- Presentation of symptoms depends upon the incubation period of species and duration of illness (Table 1).
- Early symptoms are nausea, vomiting, headache, double vision and other neurological symptoms.
- Gastroenteritis is the most common finding with abdominal cramps and diarrhea. Significant fluid and electrolyte abnormalities may occur especially in children or elderly patients.
- Metabolic acidosis or loss of bicarbonates may occur.

Table 1.   Summary of bacterial food poisoning

Organism/Species	Incubation period	Duration	Common foods affected
Staphylococcus	1–6 hrs.	2–5 days	Meats, dairy products and bakery foods
Clostridium perfringens	8–12 hrs.	24 hrs.	Meats, meat by-products especially cooked and inadequately refrigerated
Bacillus cereus	10–12 hrs.	20–36 hrs.	Reheated fried rice
Salmonella	8–40 hrs	2–5 days	Meat, dairy products, bakery foods
Campylobacter jejuni	1–7 days	1–7 days	Unpasteurized milk, dairy products
Shigella	12–50 hrs.	4–7 days	Water, fruits, vegetables
Escherichia coli (invasive)	6–36 hrs.	1–3 weeks	–
E. coli (toxigenic)	12–72 hrs.	1–2 weeks	Water

Diagnosis

Diagnosis is based on history of ingested substance and the time of onset of symptoms will help elucidate pathogens.

Laboratory/Monitoring

- Monitor CBC.
- Microscopic stool examination may demonstrate leukocytes, bacteria or presence of blood suggesting an invasive bacterial presence.
- Cultures of food, vomitus or stool may help identify pathogens.
- Monitor electrolytes, BUN, and creatinine.

Management

Pre-hospital

- Repetitive vomiting and diarrhea eliminate the need for decontamination.

Hospital

- Treatment is supportive and symptomatic.
- Diagnosis of invasive versus non-invasive bacterial diarrhea is sufficient to direct treatment.
- Fluid resuscitation is useful for patients with severe dehydration and shock.
- Treat hypotension with IV fluids and give vasopressors if needed. Norepinephrine may be added for refractory hypotension.
- Use of antidiarrheal agents is controversial though slowing of gastrointestinal activity will offer some relief for uncontrollable diarrhea, but it will also prolong the amount of time the bacteria and toxin are in contact with intestinal mucosa.
- In patients with invasive bacterial infection, antibiotics may be used once the stool culture reveals the presence of specific bacteria responsible. Empirical treatment with ciprofloxacin or trimethoprim-sulfamethoxazole is commonly given while awaiting culture results.
- There is no role for enhanced removal procedures.
- There is no specific antidote.

11. Botulism

It is a potentially life-threatening paralytic condition caused by the neurotoxins produced by *Clostridium botulinum*. *C. botulinum* is an aerobic spore-forming, gram positive rod and it produces a potent exotoxin. Five different types of clinical botulism are observed. (a) Foodborne botulism is produced by the ingestion of preformed toxin in the contaminated food. Germination of spores in food is enhanced when the pH is > 4.5, sodium chloride concentration is less than 3.5% or a low nitrite level. (b) Infant botulism is produced by the *in vivo* production of the toxin in the immature infant gut. (c) Wound botulism is observed in intravenous drug abusers and also from infected wounds. It shows clinical evidence of botulism following trauma, with a resultant infected wound and no history suggestive of foodborne illness. (d) Infant type adult botulism is produced by the intestinal colonization of *C. botulinum* and *in vivo* production of the toxin where the patients often have a history of abdominal surgery, achlorhydria, Crohn's disease or recent antibiotic treatment. (e) Inadvertent botulism may be produced when patients are treated with intramuscular injections of botulinum toxin. Purified botulinum toxin is used in the treatment of strabismus, blepharospasm, spasmodic dysphonia, hemifacial spasm, specific dystonia and other movement disorders.

Mechanism of toxicity
The toxin binds irreversibly to cholinergic nerve terminals and prevents acetylcholine release from the axon.

Toxic dose
Contaminated food containing 0.05 μg of toxin may be fatal.

Clinical effects

Foodborne botulism

- Nausea, vomiting, abdominal cramps or diarrhea are the initial symptoms.
- Constipation, dry mouth, blurred vision, and diplopia are usually the earliest neurologic symptoms.

- Dysphonia, dysarthria, dysphagia, and peripheral muscle weakness may be noted.
- Symmetric descending paralysis is a classic feature of botulism.

Wound botulism

- The clinical effects are similar to those seen in foodborne botulism except for the GI symptoms.
- The incubation period is longer which ranges from 4 to 14 days.

Infant botulism

- Constipation, progressive weakness and poor feeding are observed.
- The infant is afebrile and has a weak cry, has either absent or diminished spontaneous movements, decreased suckling, floppy head and motor response to stimuli.
- Dry mucous membranes, urinary retention, diminished GI motility, fluctuation of heart rate and changes in skin colour may also be observed.

Infant type adult botulism

- Clinical features are similar to that of infant botulism.
- The disease may simulate a Guillain-Barré Syndrome.

Inadvertent botulism

- Marked clinical weakness as well as electrophysiologic abnormalities may be observed.

Diagnosis

Diagnosis is based on classical features with a history of ingestion of home canned food, *in vivo* production of the toxin in the infant gut, IV drug abuse or infected surgical wounds, *in vivo* production of the toxin in patients with abnormal GI flora or the therapeutic use of botulinum toxin. It is confirmed by the laboratory evidence of toxin in the serum.

Laboratory/Monitoring

- Determine the toxin in the serum, stool or wound.
- Monitor electrolytes, blood sugar and arterial blood gases and electromyogram.
- Evaluate CSF if CNS infection is suspected.

Management

Pre-hospital

- Induce emesis in case of recent substantial ingestion of known or suspected contaminated material.

Hospital

- Provide symptomatic and supportive care.
- Maintain the airway and assist ventilation as required.
- Perform gastric lavage in suspected recent ingestions and in pediatric cases.
- Administer activated charcoal and cathartic in recent ingestions. Magnesium containing cathartics are contraindicated as these may depress neuromuscular conduction.

Foodborne botulism

- Administer botulin antitoxin.
- Give guanidine as adjunctive therapy to enhance release of acetylcholine at the nerve terminals which improves ocular and limb paralysis but not respiratory paralysis.

Wound botulism

- Perform surgical debridement.
- Effectiveness of antibiotics is not well proved.
- Efficacy of antitoxin is not well established.

Infant botulism

- Provide symptomatic and supportive care which is the mainstay of therapy.
- Botulin antitoxin is usually not indicated in infant botulism.

Infant type adult botulism

- Antitoxin is usually not indicated.

12. Therapeutic Drugs and Antidotes

Drug/Antidote	Indication	Dose	Comments
Activated charcoal	Variety of drugs and toxins	A: 30–100 g orally, mixed with water or sorbitol. C: 15–30 g orally Multiple dose: 0.25–0.5 g/kg every 4–6 hrs. orally or by gastric tube.	Do not give cathartic with every dose of activated charcoal in repeat dose therapy. Administer a minimum of 240 ml of diluent per 100 g of charcoal.
Antivenin	Snake bite	Sensitivity Test 0.02–0.03 ml (1:10) dilution, ID with a control test of normal saline (NS) on opposite extremity. Five reconstituted vials (1 vial diluted to 10 ml with NS) are mixed with 500 ml of NS. Administer as an IV infusion at a slow rate of 1ml/min, increase slowly to a maximum of 120 ml/hr or as tolerated. Total dose should be given in the first 4–6 hrs. Additional 5–10 vials are given depending upon the severity of envenomation. Adjust the volume of diluent depending upon the size of the patient.	Administer ASV in an ICU set up with resuscitation equipment and all emergency drugs available. Vials are rolled between hands while reconstituting. Do not shake. Positive skin reaction within 3-5 min. includes rash, flushing, anxiety. In case of positive reaction, administer IV diphenhydramine (1 mg/kg) slowly. Dilute antivenin to 1:1000 and administer under close observation. Serum sickness usually occurs within 5-44 days and is presented with fever, edema, arthralgia, nausea, vomiting, pain and muscle weakness.

Drug/Antidote	Indication	Dose	Comments
Atropine	Organophosphates Carbamates	**A:** 2–5 mg IV, slowly every 10–20 min. **C:** 0.05 mg/kg IV, slowly. The dose may be doubled every 5–10 min. until full atropinization is achieved.In cases where prolonged treatment is required, an initial bolus dose is followed by continuous infusion at the rate of 0.02–0.08 mg/kg/hr.	Full atropinization (FA) is indicated by clearing of rales and drying of pulmonary secretions. Pupillary dilation and tachycardia are not good indicators of FA. Give after maximal oxygenation in presence of cyanosis.
BAL	Copper Arsenic Mercury	**A:** 3–5 mg/kg every 4–6 hrs. by deep IM injection for first 2 days and then every 12 hrs. for 7–10 days or until recovery. **C:** 3–5 mg/kg/dose by deep IM injection every 4 hrs. for 2 days, then every 4–6 hrs. for an additional 2 days, and then every 4–12 hrs. for 7 days.	Monitor BP, HR and quantitative urine analysis for arsenic, mercury during therapy. Children on BAL may get persistent hyperpyrexia. Do not give in hepatic insufficiency except in arsenic poisoning. Do not give in patients who are allergic to peanuts or peanut products. Give in severely symptomatic patients or who can not take oral chelators in mercury poisoning.
Botulin antitoxin	Botulism	1–2 vials IV every 4 hrs. for 4–5 doses (established diagnosis). 1–2 vials given empirically. (suspected diagnosis)	Perform skin test prior to administration. IM route is not recommended.

(Contd.)

Drug/Antidote	Indication	Dose	Comments
Calcium chloride	Sodium fluoroacetate	**A:** 10–20 ml (10%) IV **C:** 10–20 mg/kg	
Calcium gluconate	Acids	**A:** 10–20 ml (10%) IV, slowly **C:** 0.2–0.3 ml/kg (10%) IV, slowly	Rapid IV administration causes hypotension, bradycardia, syncope and cardiac arrhythmias.
	Sodium fluoroacetate	**A and C > 12 yrs.** 10 ml of a 10% soln. IV slowly To be repeated as needed. **C < 12 yrs.** 200–500 mg/kg/24 hrs. (every 6 hrs. in divided doses)	
	Cardiac arrest	**A:** 100 mg/kg/dose To be repeated as needed.	
Cholestyramine	Organochlorines Yellow oleander	**A:** 4 g orally in fruit juice every 6 hrs. before meals.	May be given for several days or months.
Cyanide antidote kit (i) Amyl nitrite	Cyanide	Crush 1–2 ampules in gauze and place under the nose of the victim, who should inhale deeply for 30 secs. and repeat. Each ampule lasts for 2–3 min. If respiratory support is provided to the victim, place the ampules in the face mask or post access to the endotracheal tube.	To be continued till IV administration of sodium nitrite is started.
(ii) Sodium nitrite		**A:** 300 mg (10 ml of 3% soln.) IV over 3–5 min. **C:** 0.15–0.33 ml/kg Max.: 10 ml.	If anemia is suspected or hypotension is present, start with the lower dose, dilute in 50–100 ml of NS and administer over 5 min.

Drug/Antidote	Indication	Dose	Comments
		Pediatric dosing should be based on Hb concentration | Hb(g/dl)	Initial dose of 3% sod. nitrite (ml/kg) | |---|---| | 1 | 0.19 | | 2 | 0.25 | | 3 | 0.27 | | 4 | 0.30 | | 5 | 0.33 | | 6 | 0.36 | | 7 | 0.39 | Repeat dose: In case of no response within 30 min., an additional half of dose should be given.	Nitrite should not be administered if symptoms are mild or if the diagnosis is uncertain. Oxidation of hemoglobin to methemoglobin occurs in 30 min.
(iii) Sodium thiosulphate		A: 12.5 g (50ml, 25% solution), IV C: 1.65 ml/kg (25% solution), IV	Thiosulphate is relatively benign and may be given empirically if the diagnosis is uncertain.
Diazepam	Convulsions	A: 5–10 mg IV, slowly over 2–3 min. Max. Rate: 5 mg/min. Repeat every 10–15 min. Max.: 30 mg.	Give undiluted. Monitor BP and respiration. May be given by rectal route if IV administration is not possible.

(Contd.)

Drug/Antidote	Indication	Dose	Comments
	Anxiety/agitation	C: > 5 yrs, 1–2 mg, IV slowly over 2–3 min. Max. total dose: 10 mg. < 5 yrs, 0.2–0.5 mg IV slowly over 2–3 min. Max. total dose: 5mg.	
		0.1–0.2 mg/kg, IV initially (Max Rate: 5 mg/min. in adults and over 3 min. in children). Repeat every 1–4 hrs. as needed. Oral dose: 0.1–0.3 mg/kg.	
Diphenhydramine	Insect bites Snake bites	A: 50 mg, IV/IM C: 0.5–1 mg/kg	Excessive doses may cause flushing, tachycardia, blurred vision, delirium, toxic psychosis, urinary retention and respiratory depression.
		A: 25–50 mg, orally 6–8 hrly C: 5 mg/kg/day orally in divided doses.	In snake bites if ASV is used in a patient with + ve skin test, pretreat with IV diphenhydramine.
DMPS	Mercury Cobalt Lead Zinc Copper	5 mg/kg (5% soln.) IM or SC, 3–4 times daily during the first 24 hrs, twice or thrice on day 2 and once or twice daily on subsequent days.	Enhances urinary elimination of lead, zinc, copper and mercury.

Drug/Antidote	Indication	Dose	Comments
DMSA	Copper, Lead Arsenic Mercury	Approved only for use in children. **A:** 30 mg/kg/day in 3 divided doses for 5 days followed by 20 mg/kg/day in 2 divided doses for 14 days. **C:** Initial dose is 10 mg/kg or 350 mg/m^2 every 8 hrs. for 5 days. The dosing interval is then increased to every 12 hrs. for the next 14 days. Repeat course may be given if indicated by elevated blood lead levels. A minimum of 2 wks. between courses is recommended. The capsule contents may be administered mixed in a small amount of food.	Monitor liver function tests before therapy and then at two weeks. Side effects include rashes, nausea, vomiting, diarrhea. It may be used following EDTA and/or BAL after an interval of 4 wks.
Dopamine	Hypotension	4–6 µg/kg/min, IV	Decrease rate of administration if ventricular arrhythmias occur. Add norepinephrine if more than 20 µg/kg/min of dopamine is needed. In case of extravasation, infiltrate the affected area with phentolamine (A: 5–10 mg in 10–15 ml of NS, C: 0.1–0.2 mg/kg, Max: 10 mg with fine hypodermic needle).
	Lithium elimination	**A:** 2 µg/kg/min (based on case study)	Dose not well established Presence of optimal saline loading is required.

(Contd.)

Drug/Antidote	Indication	Dose	Comments
D-Penicillamine	Copper Mercury Lead Arsenic	**A:** 250 mg, orally 4 times a day half-an-hour before meals for 5 days or 20–40 days depending upon severity. **C:** 20 mg/kg/day, orally in two divided doses daily before meals. Max.: 1 g/day in 4 doses.	Avoid in patients with penicillin allergy. Monitor WBC counts, platelet counts, renal functions. Hypersensitivity reactions include leucopenia, thrombocytopenia, nausea, vomiting, diarrhea, renal and hepatic injury.
Doxapram	Barbiturates Severe poisoning with respiratory depression	1.5–4 mg/min., IV infusion	Not indicated in children
Epinephrine	Snake bite, wasps & bee sting Pyrethrins & Pyrethroids	0.5 ml (1:1000) SC 1:10000 for IV	To treat anaphylactic reactions
Ethyl alcohol	Methanol Ethylene glycol	IV doses of 10% soln.: Loading dose: 7.5 ml/kg Maintenance dose: 1–2 ml/kg/hr. During hemodialysis: 175–250 mg/kg/hr. Oral doses of 50% soln.: Loading dose: 1.5 ml/kg Maintenance dose: 0.2–0.4 ml/kg/hr. Maintenance dose during hemodialysis: 0.4–0.7 ml/kg/hr.	Maintain plasma ethanol concentration of 100 mg/dl Serum glucose level should be monitored in order to avoid alcohol induced hypoglycemia. Chronic alcoholics may require upto 50% higher doses of ethanol.

Drug/Antidote	Indication	Dose	Comments
Flumazenil	Benzodiazepines	**A:** 0.2 mg (2 ml) administered over 30 sec, IV. Repeat at 20 min. intervals. No more than 1mg given at any one time and not more than 3 mg in an hour except in profound coma. **C:** 10 μg/kg, IV for 2 doses.	It is associated with dizziness, facial erythema, anxiety, headache, complete heart block. It may unmask seizures in epileptic patients who are on BDZs. If patient does not respond even upto 5 mg, revise the diagnosis. Contraindicated in patients of suspected tricyclic antidepressant overdose.
Folic acid	Methanol Ethylene glycol	**A:** 50 mg IV, every 4 hrs. for 6 doses. **C:** 1 mg/kg.	It is an adjunctive treatment for methanol poisoning. May be given in ethylene glycol poisoning also. The dose mentioned here for methanol and ethylene glycol poisoning is not well established.
Fuller's earth & Bentonite	Paraquat	1–2 g/kg of fuller's earth in a 15% (w/v) aqueous suspension or 1–2 g/kg of Bentonite in a 7% (w/v) aqueous slurry.	Give adsorbent with a cathartic like magnesium sulphate (20%), mannitol or sorbitol (70%).
Furosemide	Aluminium phosphide	**A:** Low dose 20–40 mg, IV	May be tried for pulmonary edema if systolic BP > 90 mmHg. Contraindicated in the face of severe shock.
	Lithium	**A:** 10–40 mg, IV	

(Contd.)

Drug/Antidote	Indication	Dose	Comments
	Cholecalciferol	**A:** 40–120 mg, orally daily **C:** 1–2 mg/kg, orally daily, 0.5–1 mg/kg IV	Monitor serum potassium and administer KCl in case of hypokalemia.
	Barbiturates	Upto 250 mg in 25 ml (3–4 mg/min.) with sodium bicarbonate 1.4% as IV drip.	
Glucose	Hypoglycemia	**A:** 50–100 ml (50%), IV **C:** 2–4 ml/kg (25%), IV Repeat bolus of 50% in adults and 25% in children and infusion of 5–10% titrated as needed for persistent hypoglycemia.	Do not give 50% dextrose in children.
Guanidine	Botulism	15–50 mg/kg/day in 4–5 divided doses	Adjunctive therapy.
Haloperidol	Cannabis	5–10 mg, IM/IV	To treat psychotic features.
Hydroxocobalamin	Cyanide	Administer 50 times the amount of cyanide exposure. 4 g, IV in 5% dextrose. Repeat in cases of massive exposure (if the amount of cyanide exposure is unknown). Coadminister 4–8 g sodium thiosulphate.	Allergic reactions, orange red discoloration of skin, mucous membranes and urine last for 12 hrs.
Isoproterenol	*Torsade de pointes*	**A:** 2–10 µg/min. **C:** 0.1–1 µg/kg/min., continuous IV infusion	Correction of hypovolemia is recommended before infusion. Avoid simultaneous use of epinephrine. Contraindicated in acute cardiac ischaemia.

Drug/Antidote	Indication	Dose	Comments
Leucovorin	Methanol	1 mg/kg (upto 50 mg) IV, 4 hrly. for 1–2 doses followed by oral folic acid 1mg/kg (upto 50mg) 4 hrly. till the symptoms resolve.	Side effects include allergic reactions, rarely sensitization, pyrexia after parenteral administration.
Lidocaine	Tricyclic antidepressants Yellow oleander	**A:** 1 mg/kg, IV bolus over 1 min. and subsequent infusion of 1–4 mg/kg (20–50 μg/kg/min). The dose of 0.5 mg/kg, IV may be repeated at 10 min. interval if required (Max.: 300 mg or 3 mg/kg).	Serum lidocaine concentration should not exceed 1.5–5 mg/L.
Magnesium sulphate	Cathartic in various poisonings Aluminium phosphide	**A:** 20–30 g/dose, orally **C:** 250 mg/kg/dose, orally 3 g, IV bolus followed by 6 g in 12 hr. for 5–7 days	Used as a membrane stabilizing agent. Role in aluminium phosphide poisoning is controversial.
	Barium carbonate	250 mg/kg, orally	May help in precipitating barium as the insoluble sulphate salt.
	Torsade de pointes	**A:** 2 g (16 mEq) mixed in 50–100 ml 5% dextrose in water, IV over 5 min. Second dose may be repeated as needed (2 g bolus and infusion of 3–50 mg/min.) **C:** 25–50 mg/kg diluted to 10 mg/ml for IV infusion over 5–15 min.	Dose is not well established. Avoid high doses and exercise caution in renal insufficiency.
Mannitol	Fluid retention	0.5 g/kg	

(Contd.)

Drug/Antidote	Indication	Dose	Comments
Methylene blue	Methemoglobinaemia Carbon monoxide, Nitrites, Nitrates, Nitrobenzene, Copper, Dapsone	**A & C:** 1–2 mg/kg dose (0.1–0.2 ml/kg of 1% soln.) IV, slowly over 5 min. followed immediately by 15–30 ml. Fluid flush minimizes local pain and is effective and relatively safe. May be repeated in 30–60 min.	Do not repeat after two doses. Consider G-6-PD deficiency. Doses greater than 15 mg/kg may cause hemolysis. Do not use for methemoglobinemia due to sodium nitrite overdose in cyanide poisoning as cyanide will be released. Dapsone poisoning requires dosing every 6–8 hrs. for 2–3 days.
N-Acetylcysteine	Paracetamol	**A & C:** Loading dose of 140 mg/kg, orally (5% soln.) in a soft drink or water. Maintenance dose: 70 mg/kg (5%), orally every 4 hrs. for 17 doses.	Optimum efficacy within first 8–10 hrs. before metabolites of PCM accumulate. Administer slowly through a nasogastric tube to prevent vomiting. Vomiting may be prevented by high dose metoclopramide (60-70 mg, IV in adults) half-an-hour before dose. Not contraindicated in pregnancy. Contraindications: coma, vomiting, if activated charcoal is given orally.
Naloxone	Opioids	**A & C:** 0.4–2 mg (wt >20 kg). IV bolus. Repeat doses: 0.4–2 mg every 2–3 min. as needed till normal respiratory rate is achieved. Neonates may be given 10-30 μg/kg, IV.	If total dose of 10-15 mg does not produce any response, diagnosis may be questioned. With long acting opioids, a continuous infusion may be employed.

Drug/Antidote	Indication	Dose	Comments
		Children between neonates and 5 yr.: 0.1 mg/kg, IV. Maintenace: 2/3rd of the initial bolus, IV on an hrly basis at a rate of 100 ml/hr. (one half of the initial bolus dose should be readministered 15 min. after initiation of the continuous infusion to prevent drop in naloxone levels).	
Neostigmine	Snake bite	0.5–2 mg, IV at intervals of half an hour preceded by atropine A: (0.4–1.25 mg) C: 0.01–0.04 mg/kg, IM/IV	Has been used successfully to reverse muscular paralysis due to cobra neurotoxin.
Nifedipine	Scorpion sting	A: 10–20 mg, orally or sublingually, C: 5 mg C: (< 10 kg) 2.5 mg, sublingually or 0.25–0.5 mg/kg, orally	Oral administration is superior to sublingual or buccal administration in elderly. Hypotension may develop during initial treatment and more frequently in patients receiving β-blockers simultaneously.
Norepinephrine	Hypotension	A: 4–8 μg/min, IV C: 1–2μg/min., IV or 0.1 μg/kg/min. Increase as needed every 5–10 min.	Avoid extravasation.
Penicillin G	Mushrooms	A: PO, 300,000–1200,000 units/kg/24 hrs. divided in 4 doses A&C: IM/IV 3,00,000–10,000,00 units/kg/day in 4 divided doses for 5–10 days.	It is given only in mushrooms containing cyclopeptides.

(Contd.)

Drug/Antidote	Indication	Dose	Comments
Phenobarbital	Recurrent convulsions	**A:** 600–1200 mg or 10–20 mg/kg, IV diluted in 60 ml of NS (Rate: 25–50 mg/min.) Maintenance: 120–240 mg every 20 min. Max: 1–2 g **C:** 15–20 mg/kg, IV (Rate: 25–50 mg/min.) Maintenance: 5–10 mg/kg, every 20 min Max: 40 mg/kg	Monitor BP constantly. Monitor respiration as respiratory depression due to OPs may get aggravated by phenobarbital.
Phenytoin	Convulsions	**A:** 10–15 mg/kg, IV, slowly (Max. Rate: 50 mg/min) Maintenance: 100 mg, orally or IV every 6–8 hrs. Max: 1000 mg **C:** 15–20 mg/kg, IV, slowly (Rate: 1 mg/kg/min) Maintenance: 1.5 mg/kg every 30 min, Max: 20 mg/kg/day	Monitor BP and ECG. Stop or slow infusion in case of hypotension or arrhythmias. Avoid extravasation. Follow each injection with an infusion of sterile saline through the same needle.
Physostigmine	Datura Mushrooms Antihistamines	**A:** 0.5–2 mg, slow IV push **C:** 0.02 mg/kg Repeat every 20–30 min. as needed.	Monitor cardiac status during administration. IM or continuous IV infusion is contraindicated. Give atropine in case of excessive muscarinic stimulation.

Drug/Antidote	Indication	Dose	Comments
Phytonadione (Vitamin K₁)	Warfarin Superwarfarins NSAIDs	A: 5–10 mg, SC C: 1–5 mg, SC May be repeated in 6–8 hrs. C: 5–10 mg/day A: 10–25 mg/day	Switch to oral therapy as soon as possible for maintenance. Daily doses of 50–200 mg have been required in some cases. Therapy may be required for several weeks or even months. IM route is preferred if risk of bleeding is low. IV administration is used rarely only when hemorrhage is present or imminent depending on the severity of anticoagulation, A: 10–50 mg C: 0.6 mg/kg (< 12 yrs.) diluted in preservative free dextrose or NS. Administer slowly. Rate not to exceed 1 mg/min or 5% of the total dose per min., whichever is slower. IV infusion can cause flushing, chest pain, dyspnea and anaphylaxis.
Polyethylene glycol	Lithium	A: 1–2 L/hr. C: 25 ml/kg/hr. Continue till rectal effluent is as clear as PEG being administered.	Prolonged irrigation may lead to mild metabolic acidosis. Assess bowel motility before and during this process.
Potassium chloride	Barium carbonate	A: 0.5–1.0 mEq/min in 0.9% or 0.45% saline C: 0.3 mEq/kg/dose/hr., IV infusion	

(Contd.)

Drug/Antidote	Indication	Dose	Comments
Potassium ferric ferrocynaide (Prussian blue)	Thallium	250 mg/kg/day in 2–4 divided doses	Continue therapy till the urinary excretion of thallium is 0–10 μg/24hrs.
Pralidoxime (2-PAM)	Organophosphates Carbamates	A: 1–2 g, IV over 5–10 min mixed in 250 ml of NS and infused over 5–30 min. C: 25–50 mg/kg, diluted to 5% concentration in NS and infused over 5–30 min. This dose may be repeated after one hour. If muscle or diaphragmatic weakness and coma are not relieved, repeat this dose every 6–12 hrs. Give continuous infusion in severe poisoning A: 500 mg/hr. Max: 12 g/24 hr. C: 9–19 mg/kg/hr after an initial bolus.	Titration should be based on clinical response. Efficacy of oral pralidoxime is limited by vomiting early in the course of poisoning or by potential of adsorption to administered activated charcoal. Intravenous infusion is preferred. Presentation 24–48 hrs. post poisoning is not a contraindication to treatment with PAM. It is indicated in carbamate poisoning only in case of respiratory depression or severe muscle weakness or concomitant organophosphate and carbamate exposure.
Prazosin	Scorpion sting	0.25–0.5 mg, orally. Repeat every 4–6 hrs.	Not recommended in children.
Propranolol	Datura	A: 0.5–3 mg, IV C: 0.01–0.02 mg/kg, IV Max. dose: 1 mg/dose	Monitor heart rate and BP.
Ranitidine	GI irritation	50 mg, IV every 8 hrs.	

Drug/Antidote	Indication	Dose	Comments
Sodium bicarbonate	Metabolic acidosis	50 mEq/15 min.	Administer if arterial bicarbonate is below 15 mmol/L. Ideally total base deficit should be calculated and corrected over a period of 3–4 hrs. with the idea of restoring blood pH to near normal.
	Antihistamines Tricyclic antidepressants	A: 1–2 mEq/kg, IV bolus, May be repeated as needed (serum pH should not exceed 7.45–7.55)	Correct acidemia before administration. Monitor ABGs to avoid excessive alkelemia.
Sorbitol	Catharsis	A: 1–2 g/kg/dose, orally Max: 150 g/dose C: 1–1.5 g/kg/dose as a 35% soln., orally Max: 50 g/dose	Do not give with every dose of activated charcoal in repeat dose charcoal therapy.
Sucralfate	NSAIDs	1g, four times daily before meals for a minimum of 4 wks.	Not indicated in children
Syrup of ipecac	Emesis	A: 30 ml C: (1–2 yrs) 15 ml Infants: (6–12 months): 5–10 ml	Induces vomiting within 30 min. Administer 30 min. before charcoal. Can be given at home.

Index